Asian Paleo Cookbook

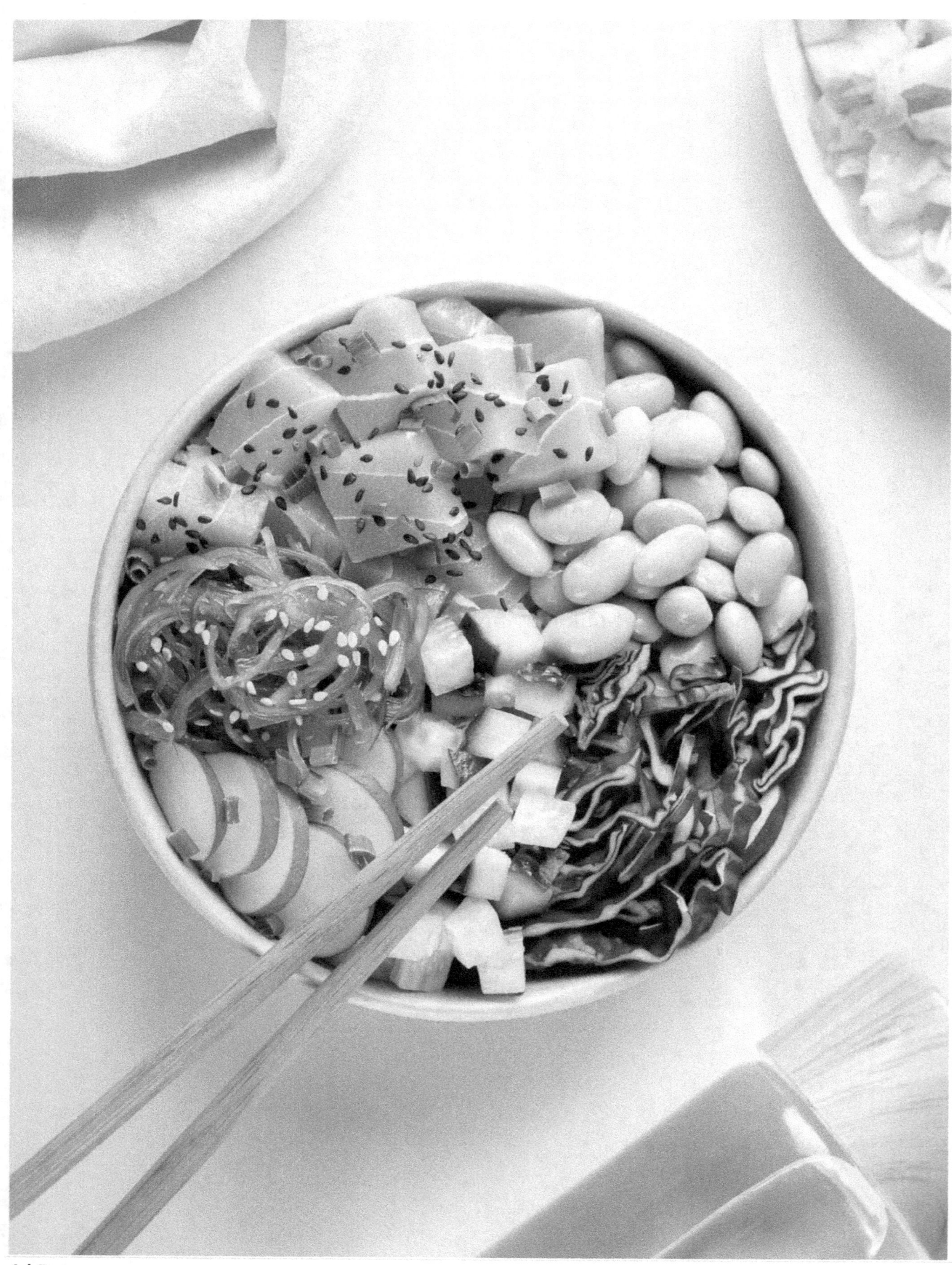

Introduction

Welcome to "Asian Paleo Cookbook"!

Meet the Author: Natalia Gerlach

Hello, young chefs and food lovers! Have you ever heard of Natalia Gerlach? She's an amazing cook who loves exploring different flavors from Asia. Amaya has a special talent for making healthy and yummy food. She knows a lot about the Paleo diet, which is all about eating natural foods like our ancestors. Natalia traveled across Asia to learn secret recipes and now, she's sharing them with us in this fantastic cookbook!

What's Inside the Book?

This book isn't just any cookbook. It's a journey through the tasty world of Paleo with an Asian twist. Natalia has put together 120 recipes that are both delicious and good for you.

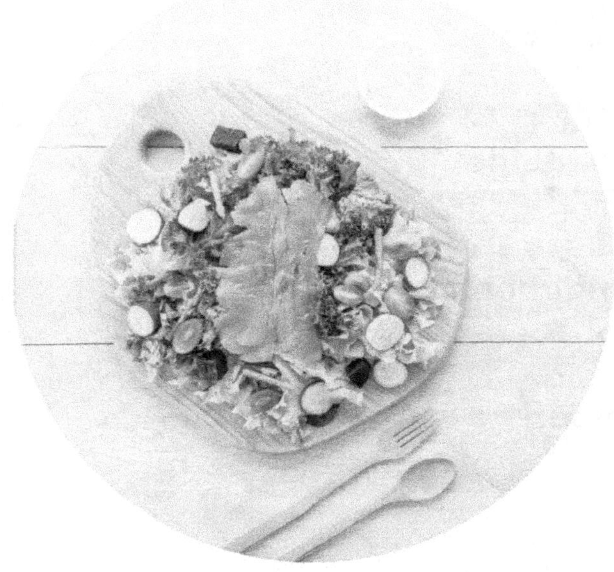

Chapters

Why You'll Love This Cookbook?

"Asian Paleo Cookbook" is more than just a collection of recipes. It's a treasure trove of new tastes, healthy eating, and fun cooking experiences. Natalia Gerlach makes sure that each recipe is easy to follow and exciting to cook. This book is perfect for young chefs who want to explore new flavors while keeping their meals healthy and yummy.

Whether you're cooking for yourself, your friends, or your family, these recipes will bring smiles to everyone's faces. So, are you ready to embark on a delicious adventure with Natalia Gerlach? Your kitchen awaits!

Explore, Cook, and Enjoy!

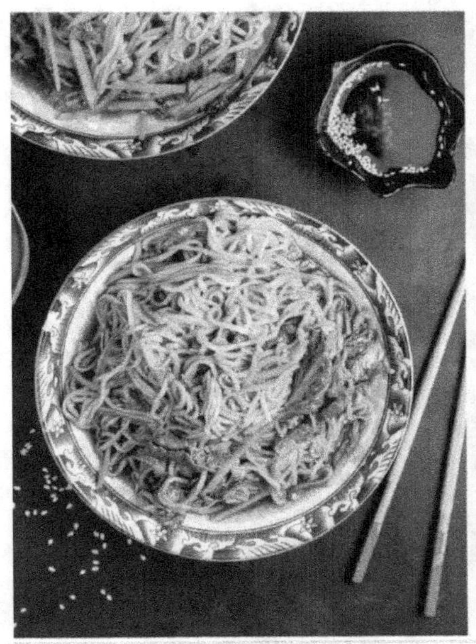
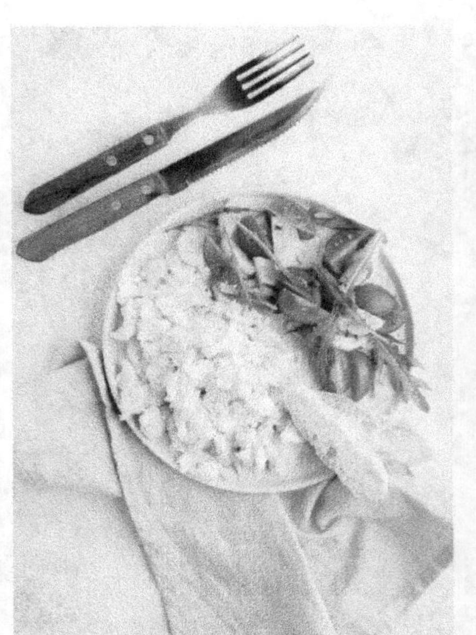
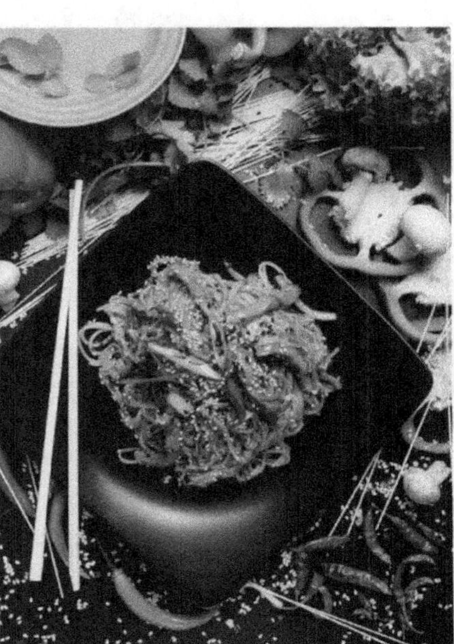

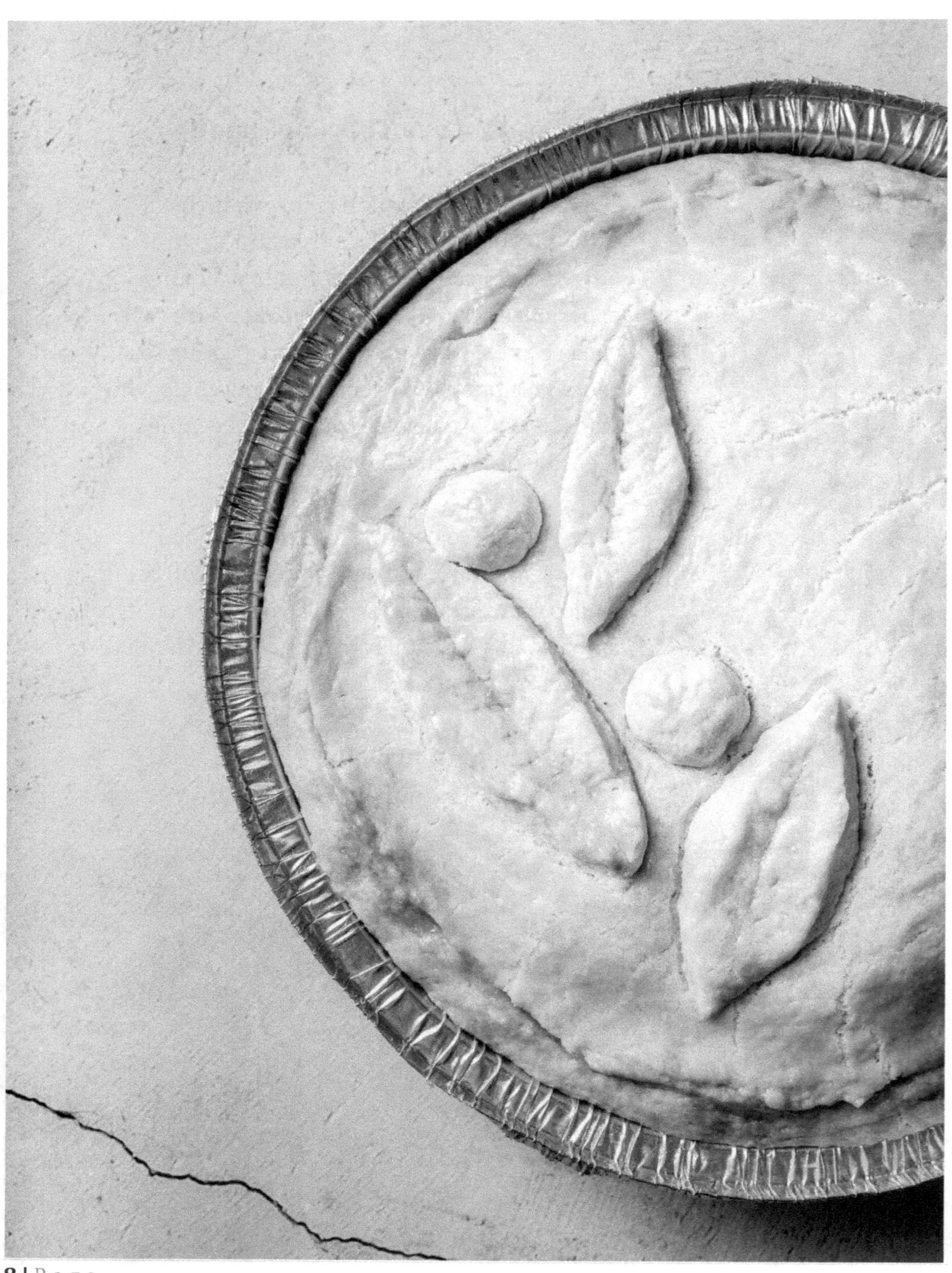

Table Of Content

01. FLUFFY VEGAN SCRAMBLED EGGS

Prep Time: 6 Hours 10 Minutes | Cook Time: 5 Minutes

Total Time: 6 Hours 15 Minutes | Serving: 6

Ingredients

- 3/4 tsp ground turmeric
- 1 ¼ tsp baking powder
- 1 ⅓ cup of canned light coconut milk
- 1/2 tsp onion powder
- 2 Tbsp olive or avocado oil
- 1/4 cup of white rice flour
- 3/4 cup of split mung beans, rinsed
- 2 tsp nutritional yeast
- 1 – 1 ¼ tsp black salt

Instructions

1. Rinse mung beans and mix in a large bowl. Cover with lukewarm water and soak overnight or at least 6 hours.
2. First, drain and rinse, then blend on high. Combine remaining ingredients and blend until smooth. Taste and add black salt for "eggy" flavor, onion powder, turmeric, or nutritional yeast for cheesiness. The batter should be thin and pourable but not watery. Increase rice flour or coconut milk if it is too thin or thick.
3. Heat a nonstick pan (we love this one) or greased skillet over medium-low heat. Add 1/4 cup of (60 g) egg mixture to the pan when hot, almost to the edges. Then cover.
4. Cook until edges are dry, 1-2 minutes. Surface bubbles may appear. Then, gently push the "eggs" to one side of the pan with a rubber spatula. Cover and cook another 1-2 minutes.
5. Eat them as "soft scrambled eggs" or cook longer. Flip to cook the top better.
6. Transfer the egg to a plate and cool slightly. Taste cooked egg and adjust batter flavor as needed, adding black salt for "eggy" flavor or to hide baking powder flavor.
7. Thoroughly cook the egg mixture! Store in the fridge for a week to use throughout.
8. This mixture works well for scrambled eggs, but sautéing onion, garlic, veggies, or greens before adding it may work too.
9. Serve plain or with salsa, vegan parmesan cheese, fresh herbs, or toast.

02. SWEET POTATO & SPROUT HASH WITH POACHED EGGS

Prep Time: 15 Minutes | Cook Time: 25 Minutes | Total Time: 40 Minutes | Serving: 3

Ingredients

- grating of nutmeg
- 3 eggs
- 2 large sweet potatoes, cut into chunks
- 2 red onions, thinly sliced
- 2 tsp olive oil
- 300g brussels sprouts, thinly sliced

Instructions

1. Cover the sweet potatoes with food wrap in a bowl and microwave on high for 5 minutes until tender but still firm. Uncover and cool the bowl.
2. Meanwhile, heat oil in a wide nonstick pan and add onions. Cook for 5-8 minutes to caramelize. Add sprouts and stir-fry on high until softened. After pushing the Brussels sprouts and onions to one side, add the sweet potatoes and squash them with a spatula. Leave it unattended for 5 minutes to crisp the underside. Season, add nutmeg, mix in sprouts and onions, and flip the potato without breaking it up. Cook for 5 more minutes to crisp.
3. Meanwhile, poach 3 eggs in barely simmering water. Serve poached eggs on hash.

03. SPINACH BLUEBERRY BANANA SMOOTHIE

Prep Time: 5 Minutes | Cook Time: 5 Minutes | Total Time: 10 Minutes | Serving:

Ingredients

- ½ cup of blueberries
- 1 banana ripe, frozen even better
- 1 ½ cup of spinach fresh, about 2.5ounce
- 1 cup of soy milk
- 6 ice cubes
- ⅛ tsp pumpkin spice mix

Optional (recommended):

- 2 tbsp Organic Protein Plant-Based Powder
- ¼ cup of oatmeal
- 1 tbsp date paste

Instructions

1. Add dairy-free milk to the blender first, then the spinach and frozen foods.
2. It takes about 40 seconds to blend until smooth.Serve right away.

04. STEAK AND EGGS

Prep Time: 5 Minutes | Cook Time: 15 Minutes

Total Time: 20 Minutes | Serving: 2

Ingredients

- 4 large Eggs
- 1 tsp Sea salt
- 1 tsp Black pepper
- Chopped parsley
- 2 tbsp Avocado oil
- 1 8-oz Sirloin steak

Instructions

1. Using paper towels, pat the steak dry on both sides. Sprinkle ½ tsp of sea salt and ¼ tsp of black pepper over both sides.
2. Set a cast-iron skillet with medium heat and add 1 tbsp of avocado oil.
3. With great care, place the steak in the skillet. Quickly remove from pan after 60 to 90 seconds of searing one side. Unless it becomes easily removable, cook it until it does. After 1 minute, flip the steak. Flip the steak every 60-90 seconds for an additional 4 minutes. Sear the steak for 6 minutes or until it reaches a medium-rare doneness, depending on your preference.
4. If you want your steak rare, medium rare, medium, or well done, use a meat thermometer and set the temperature to 120 degrees Fahrenheit (49 degrees Celsius). Once heated, place a layer of aluminum foil over it. To get a 5-degree internal temperature increase in the steak, let it rest for 10 minutes before slicing.
5. Meanwhile, heat a medium nonstick skillet on low. Crack all 4 eggs carefully into the pan with the remaining 1 tbsp of avocado oil—season with remaining salt (⅛ tsp per egg) and pepper (1/16 tsp per egg). Lid the pan and cook over low heat until the whites set.
6. Cut the steak in half for two 4-ounce servings. Strip against the grain and serve with fried eggs. Add fresh parsley if desired.

05. PALEO ALMOND BUTTER COOKIES

Prep Time: 10 Minutes | Cook Time: 10 Minutes

Total Time: 20 Minutes | Serving: 16

Ingredients

- 1 tsp baking soda
- 1 large egg, room temperature
- 1 cup of coconut sugar
- 1 cup of almond butter or store-bought works, too, room temperature
- 1 tsp pure vanilla extract

Instructions

1. Set the oven to 350º with two racks in the center place. Cover two baking sheets with parchment or silpat.
2. Stir all ingredients in a medium bowl.
3. Use a cookie scoop to scoop 1.5 tbsp balls of dough onto the baking sheet with room to spread.
4. Bake for 9-10 minutes to set edges and puff centers. Cookies flatten and "crackle" when cooled. Let cool for 10 minutes, and enjoy! It pairs well with homemade almond milk.
5. Cookies last a week in an airtight container or a year in the freezer.

06. GREEN SHAKSHUKA

Prep Time: 10 Minutes | Cook Time: 25 Minutes

Total Time: 35 Minutes | Serving: 4

Ingredients

- ¼ tsp sea salt, more to taste
- ⅓ cup of crumbled feta cheese
- 2 tbsp extra-virgin olive oil
- 3 medium garlic cloves, minced
- ¼ cup of fresh parsley leaves
- 2 tbsp harissa paste
- 1 avocado, diced
- Pinch of cayenne pepper, optional
- Microgreens for garnish, optional

- ½ tsp smoked paprika
- ½ tsp ground cumin
- 1 cup of chopped yellow onion
- 1 cup of fresh spinach, chopped
- 1 red bell pepper, seeded and diced
- Freshly ground black pepper
- 1 28-ounce can of crushed tomatoes
- 3 to 5 eggs

Instructions

1. In a 12-inch lidded stainless steel or enamel-coated cast-iron skillet, heat oil on medium. Add the onion, red pepper, salt, and several grinds of fresh pepper and cook for 6–8 minutes until soft and translucent.
2. Add garlic, paprika, cumin, and cayenne, if using, to medium-low heat. Stir and cook for 30 to 40 seconds before adding tomatoes and harissa paste. Simmer for 10 to 20 minutes to thicken the sauce.
3. Stir in spinach to wilt. Make 3–5 sauce wells with the back of a spoon. Crack eggs. Cover and cook eggs for 5–8 minutes until set. How runny you like your egg yolks determines the timing.
4. If using, add feta, parsley, avocado, and microgreens and season with salt and pepper. Offer toasted bread for scooping.

07. WHOLE30 BREAKFAST SAUSAGE

Prep Time: 5 Minutes | Cook Time: 10 Minutes

Total Time: 15 Minutes | Serving: 8

Ingredients

- 1 pound ground pork
- 2 tbsp pure lard melted
- 1/4 tsp onion powder
- 1 tsp fennel seeds
- 1 tsp dried sage
- 1/2 tsp ground black pepper
- pinch of nutmeg
- 3/4 tsp acceptable sea salt
- 1/2 tsp garlic powder
- Lard for frying

Instructions

1. Mix ground pork and 2 tbsp melted lard in a large bowl. Mix by hand.
2. Mix fennel, garlic powder, black pepper, sage, salt, and onion powder in a small bowl.
3. Sprinkle and mix the seasonings on the pork. Make 8 equal-sized pork patties.
4. I was frying pan with 1-2 Tbsp lard. Add sausage patties (cook in batches if needed) to the hot pan and cook for 5 minutes per side until cooked and no longer pink in the middle.

09. PALEO NUT ENERGY BARS

Prep Time: 10 Minutes | Cook Time: 17 Minutes | Total Time: 27 Minutes | Serving: 16

Ingredients

- 1 1/2 tsp vanilla
- 1 cup of chopped walnuts
- 2 tbsp cinnamon
- 20 dates finely chopped
- 1 cup of chopped almonds
- 2 cups of chopped pecans
- 3/4 cup of egg whites

Instructions

1. Preheat the oven to 350.
2. Mix all ingredients in a large bowl.
3. Line the 9x13 pan with parchment or aluminum foil and spray with cooking spray. Press the nut mixture into the pan bottom.
4. Bake 16-18 minutes. Pull the wax paper to remove the bars from the pan after 5 minutes of cooling. Slice the bars into desired rectangles with a pizza cutter.

08. HEARTY PALEO SWEET POTATO BREAD

Prep Time: 15 Minutes | Cook Time: 1 Hour

Total Time: 1 Hour 15 Minutes | Serving: 14

Ingredients

- 3 Tbsp coconut flour
- 5 tbsp organic coconut oil melted
- 1/2 tsp plus a pinch of fine-grain sea salt
- 1/4 cup of tapioca flour
- 1 tsp pure maple syrup
- 1 cup of + 5 Tbsp blanched almond flour
- 4 large eggs
- 1 tsp baking soda
- 1 tbsp raw apple cider vinegar
- 1/2 cup of mashed sweet potato

Instructions

1. Set your oven to 350 degrees and line a medium 8 x 4 loaf pan*** with parchment paper.
2. Mix eggs and mashed sweet potato in a large bowl until smooth. Stir in coconut oil, honey or maple, and vinegar (don't overbeat).
3. Blend almond, coconut, and tapioca flours, baking soda, and salt in a medium bowl.
4. Avoid overmixing the batter by slowly adding the dry ingredients until just moistened.
5. Lift the batter with a rubber spatula into the parchment-lined loaf pan and bake for 1 hour in the preheated oven (check around 50 minutes for a nicely browned top and a clean toothpick).
6. After 10 minutes in the loaf pan, transfer the loaf to a wire rack with both sides of parchment paper and cool for 1-2 hours before slicing.
7. Refrigerate leftovers in plastic or parchment paper, and enjoy! This bread goes well with nut butter, pastured butter, eggs, and sandwiches.

09. PALEO NUT ENERGY BARS

Prep Time: 10 Minutes | Cook Time: 17 Minutes

Total Time: 27 Minutes | Serving: 16

Ingredients

- 1 1/2 tsp vanilla
- 1 cup of chopped walnuts
- 2 tbsp cinnamon
- 20 dates finely chopped
- 1 cup of chopped almonds
- 2 cups of chopped pecans
- 3/4 cup of egg whites

Instructions

5. Preheat the oven to 350.
6. Mix all ingredients in a large bowl.
7. Line the 9x13 pan with parchment or aluminum foil and spray with cooking spray. Press the nut mixture into the pan bottom.
8. Bake 16-18 minutes. Pull the wax paper to remove the bars from the pan after 5 minutes of cooling. Slice the bars into desired rectangles with a pizza cutter.

10. SHEET PAN CHICKEN AND ASPARAGUS

Prep Time: 10 Minutes | Cook Time: 15 Minutes | Total Time: 35 Minutes | Serving: 4

Ingredients

- ¾ tsp Freshly ground black pepper divided
- 1 tbsp avocado oil
- 1½ tsp Diamond Crystal kosher salt divided
- 1 tbsp arrowroot powder
- 3 garlic cloves minced
- 2 tbsp coconut aminos
- ½ tbsp minced fresh ginger
- 2 tsp toasted sesame seeds, optional garnish
- 2pounds boneless, skinless chicken thighs
- 2 tsp lime zest
- 2 tbsp Red Boat fish sauce
- 2 tsp toasted sesame oil
- 3 tbsp full-fat coconut milk
- 2 tbsp lime juice
- 1 pound asparagus tough ends trimmed
- 3 tbsp honey
- 2 tbsp fresh cilantro leaves, optional garnish
- 3 tbsp freshly squeezed orange juice

Instructions

1. When the chicken thighs are dry, cut them into 1½- to 2-inch pieces.
2. Add ½ tsp of pepper and 1 tsp of kosher salt to the chicken, then toss it well to coat it with the spices.
3. Mix orange juice, ginger, garlic, sesame oil, avocado oil, lime zest and juice, coconut milk, arrowroot powder, and fish sauce in a large bowl using a whisk.
4. Put the chicken pieces in and toss them around to cover them with the meat sauce. Let the chicken sit out at room temperature for twenty to thirty minutes. You can marinate it in the fridge up to two days ahead of time, but instead of fresh ginger, use ground ginger.
5. Set the rack 6 inches away from the heat source and turn the broiler on high.
6. Use a little avocado oil to grease a sheet pan. Place the chicken on the sheet pan in a single layer on one side and use tongs or a slotted spoon to do this.
7. On the other side of the pan, put the asparagus. Add ¼ tsp of black pepper and ½ tsp of kosher salt to the asparagus.
8. Spread the sauce all over the chicken and asparagus.
9. For 10 to 12 minutes, stir the food every so often while cooking under the broiler. When the chicken is fully cooked, the asparagus is nicely browned, and the sauce has become a little thicker, the sheet pan is done.
10. You can add sesame seeds and cilantro as a garnish. Serve with cauliflower rice.

11. SAUSAGE EGG MUFFINS

Prep Time: 5 Minutes | Cook Time: 23 Minutes

Total Time: 28 Minutes | Serving: 12

Ingredients

- 3/4 tsp Sea salt
- 1/2 tsp Black pepper
- 8 large Eggs
- 3/4 cup of Cheddar cheese (shredded)
- 1pound Ground Italian sausage
- 1/4 cup of Heavy cream

Instructions

1. Please turn on the oven and heat it up to 400 degrees F (204 degrees C).
2. Cook the ground sausage in a large skillet over medium-high heat for 8 to 10 minutes, breaking it up with a wooden spoon as you go. It should be golden brown.
3. Line a muffin tin with 12 silicone muffin liners while you wait.
4. Put the ground sausage into the muffin tins. Add cheese on top.
5. Add the eggs, heavy cream, sea salt, and black pepper to a bowl and whisk them together. Put the sausage in the muffin cups of and then pour the egg mixture on top of it.
6. Set the eggs by baking for 15 to 20 minutes.

12. VEGETARIAN BIBIMBAP BOWL WITH BIBIMBAP SAUCE

Prep Time: 40 Minutes | Cook Time: 10 Minutes | Total Time: 50 Minutes | Serving: 4

Ingredients

- Toasted white sesame seeds, sprinkle
- 3-4 bulbs of scallions, chopped, about 1 bulb for each vegetable item
- 2-3 tsp Toasted sesame oil
- ½ tsp acceptable sea salt for each vegetable item or to taste
- 0-15ounce . spinach
- 1.5- 2 tsp grated garlic
- 1 tbsp coconut aminos
- 3 medium carrots
- 0ounce . mung bean sprouts
- 1 tsp apple cider vinegar
- ½ tsp garlic powder
- 3 medium zucchinis

Bibimbap Sauce:

- 2.5 tbsp apple cider vinegar
- 3 tbsp water
- 2.5 tbsp tomato paste
- ½ tsp onion powder
- 2-3 tsp gochugaru,
- 6 whole Medjool dates,
- 2 tbsp coconut aminos

- A little salt to taste
- 1 tsp toasted sesame oil

Other:

- Cauliflower fried rice, or steamed white
- 1-1.5 tbsp avocado oil to saute zucchini
- 4 large eggs, pan-fried sunny side up

Instructions

1. Use a mandolin slicer to cut the zucchini into slices that are just a bit thinner than ¼-inch (0.6 cm) thick. Put 1.5 tsp of acceptable sea salt on each piece and rub it in slowly. Place in a roomy space for twenty minutes or up to an hour. After pressing out the water, quickly sauté the beans with garlic, avocado oil, and sesame oil. Put sesame seeds and scallions on top. Please put it in the fridge.
2. For the spinach, mung bean sprouts, and carrots:
3. Cut up the carrots. The steps for cooking these vegetables are the same, but please cook them one at a time. Add some salt to a big pot of water and bring it to a boil. It takes two minutes for hot water to blanch carrots, two minutes for bean sprouts, and thirty seconds for spinach. Soak in cold water for a while, then squeeze out the water. Put salt, garlic, sesame oil, scallions, and sesame seeds in a large bowl. Then, season each vegetable with

them. Taste it and change how much salt you use. Could you put it in the fridge? For extra flavor, you choose to add a tbsp of coconut aminos, but you don't have to.

4. To make the bibimbap sauce, put the pieces from the dates to the salt in a small food processor. Mix it a few times to make a paste. You'll need to scrape the bowl numerous times. Put the paste in a small bowl. Put the vinegar and sesame oil and mix them in. Change the amount of vinegar to your liking.
5. To put together:
6. The cooked rice (or cauliflower rice) should go in the bottom of the bowls. Then, put a vegetable on top of the rice. I like to switch up the colors of the vegetables so they look nice. You can put a fried egg on top with the white side up, a lot of homemade bibimbap sauce, and a tsp of sesame seeds. Use a spoon to mix it all up, then eat it!

13. BANG BANG CAULIFLOWER

Prep Time: 5 Minutes | Cook Time: 10 Minutes

Total Time: 15 Minutes | Serving: 4

Ingredients

- Air Fryer Cauliflower Ingredients
- 1 head cauliflower cut into florets
- salt + pepper to taste
- 1 tbsp olive oil

Bang Bang Sauce Ingredients:

- ½ cup of Primal Kitchen Avocado Mayo
- 2 tbsp sweet Thai chili sauce
- 1 tsp rice vinegar
- 1 tbsp Sriracha sauce

Instructions

1. How to Cook Cauliflower in an Air Fryer
2. Put olive oil on the cauliflower. Add salt and pepper to taste.
3. Spray coconut oil cooking spray on the food and put it in the air fryer. For 10 minutes, cook at 400F and shake every 5 minutes.
4. How to Make Bang Bang Sauce
5. Add the sauce ingredients in a small size bowl and set them aside while the cauliflower cooks in the air fryer.
6. Put the cauliflower and bang bang sauce in a bowl after it's done cooking. Start by adding three to five tbsp of bang bang sauce, and then add more if you want. Serve right away.

14. CAULIFLOWER GNOCCHI

Prep Time: 30 Minutes | Cook Time: 20 Minutes

Total Time: 50 Minutes | Serving: 4

Ingredients

- olive oil spray
- 1 cup of white whole-wheat flour
- 2 cups of marinara sauce, jarred or homemade
- Grated Parmesan cheese for topping, optional
- 3 pounds cauliflower florets
- 1 tsp kosher salt
- Basil, optional for serving

Instructions

1. Place the cauliflower in a large pot. Add enough water to cover the vegetables. Bring the pot to a boil.
2. Turn down the heat, cover the cauliflower, and let it cook for 22 minutes until it is very soft. After draining, set it aside to cool.
3. After the cauliflower has cooled, put a third to half of it in a dish towel and squeeze out as much water as you can. Then, put the cauliflower in a large bowl. Do this again and again with the rest of the cauliflower until it is 100% drained and squeezed dry so the dough doesn't stick together too much.
4. In a bowl with the mashed cauliflower, combine the flour and salt using a fork.
5. Then, use your hands to fold and squeeze the ingredients together to make a dough.
6. Sprinkle flour on a work surface and cut the dough into 8 equal pieces, each about 2 1/2 ounces. Roll each ball into a ½-inch-thick rope that is 10 inches long and set it aside. Keep going until you've used up all the dough.
7. Next, cut each rope into 13 pieces of the same size, like gnocchi. Barely space the pieces apart so they don't touch. There should be 108 pieces in all. If the dough gets too sticky to work with, sprinkle your hands with flour.
8. Mist a big skillet with nonstick oil, spray a lot, then warm it up over medium-low heat in two batches. Put half of the gnocchi in the hot pan. If the pieces stick together, use the spatula to separate them in the pan. Put only a few things in the pan at a time, or the gnocchi will take too long to cook.
9. Leave the gnocchi in the hot pan for two minutes without moving them. Then, use a spoon or tongs to carefully flip them over without squashing them. Put salt on top, and cook for another 2 to 4 minutes or until done the way you like it.
10. Set this aside and do it again with the rest of the gnocchi. Then, put everything back in the skillet and pour the marinara over it. Stir it and serve with grated cheese on top if you want.

15. RATATOUILLE (FRENCH VEGETABLE STEW)

Prep Time: 20 Minutes | Cook Time: 60 Minutes

Total Time: 1 Hour 15 Minutes | Serving: 6

Ingredients

- 8–14 garlic cloves, whole, peeled
- 4 cups of eggplant- 3 Japanese eggplant or one large globe eggplant
- 2–3 tbsp fresh herbs – fresh thyme, oregano, rosemary, or any combination.
- 1 onion
- olive oil for drizzling
- splash balsamic vinegar or red wine vinegar
- 2 medium tomatoes
- 2 medium zucchini or yellow summer squash
- 1–2 red bell pepper – or use yellow bell pepper or green bell pepper
- salt and black pepper to taste

Instructions

1. Warm the oven up to 400F and put parchment paper on two sheet pans.
2. Get the veggies ready: You can use a vegetable peeler to peel the eggplant, or you can cut off long strips of skin. You can also leave the skin on if you'd rather. Cut into bite-sized pieces that are ½ inch thick. Cut the bell pepper into strips that are ½ inch wide. For the tomatoes, cut them into 3/4-inch wedges. Cut the zucchini in half lengthwise, then into half-moons that are ½ inch thick. Cut the onion into half-moons that are ½ inch thick.
3. Put the vegetables on the sheet pan so that they are all in one layer. You will need two sheet pans for this.
4. Add olive oil and toss, making sure there is enough oil to cover everything well. Sprinkle salt and pepper on top. Throw well.
5. Put the vegetables in a hot oven for 20 minutes. After that, add the herbs and whole, peeled garlic cloves and mix them all. After 20 minutes, remix it. Lower the heat to 300F and roast for another 10 to 20 minutes, or until the beans are soft and the edges start to turn caramelized. Pay close attention at this point.
6. Take it out of the oven, taste it, and add more salt and pepper if needed. Then, add a splash of vinegar and carefully mix it in.
7. Cool it down and put it in the fridge (or freezer) until you're ready to use it.

16. SWEET POTATO NOODLES

Prep Time: 10 Minutes | Cook Time: 30 Minutes

Total Time: 1 Hour 20 Minutes | Serving: 4

Ingredients

- 4 medium sweet potatoes
- 1 tsp ground black pepper, divided
- 1 tbsp chopped fresh parsley
- 1 tbsp vegetable bouillon
- 1 tbsp olive oil
- 1 1/2 cups of frozen spinach
- 1 tsp salt, divided
- 1 medium onion, sliced
- 1 tbsp Parmesan cheese, garnish
- 3/4 cup of water
- 2 cloves garlic, chopped
- 5 slices bacon, diced
- 1 cup of cashews

Instructions

1. Get the ingredients together.
2. Put the cashews in a bowl and add enough water to cover them. Soak for at least an hour and up to four hours.
3. Clean the sweet potatoes, then peel them.
4. Take the ends off of both sides of each sweet potato and throw them away. Put a potato on the spiral vegetable slicer's spikes.
5. To make long noodles, turn the spiral vegetable slicer and press down evenly. Do not use the noodles.
6. Turn on the medium-high heat and warm up a big, shallow saucepan. When you add the diced bacon, stir it around a lot of times so it gets crispy. Take out the bacon using a slotted spoon, but don't wipe off the grease. Keep the crispy bacon until you're ready to serve.
7. Keep the onion and olive oil in the pan. Add about half of the salt and pepper, and stir it in every so often. Cook over medium heat for about 20 minutes or until it gets soft and slightly caramelized.
8. Make the cashew sauce at the same time. Rinse and drain the cashews. Mix in a blender with 3/4 cup of water, the vegetable broth, the garlic, and the rest of the salt and pepper. Use a high-speed blender to make it smooth.
9. As the onion turns brown, add the spinach to the pan and stir it around until it's warm all the way through.
10. After you add the sweet potato noodles, stir and toss them around for about 5 minutes or until they get soft.
11. Put the Parmesan cheese on top and enjoy.

17. SPICY SPAGHETTI SQUASH NOODLES

Prep Time: 10 Minutes | Cook Time: 8 Minutes

Total Time: 18 Minutes | Serving: 4

Ingredients

- Two cans (or 27ounce) of full-fat coconut milk.
- 2-4 tbsp arrowroot flour f
- 2 tsp poultry seasoning
- 2 tsp of chopped garlic
- 2 scoops of sea salt
- 1 small white onion,
- 1/2 tsp red pepper flakes
- 1 tsp paprika

Instructions

1. Put olive oil in a spacious pan and add the chopped onions. Cook for a few minutes over medium-low heat until the onions turn golden. But don't add the arrowroot flour yet. Next, add the remaining sauce ingredients and stir. First, bring the sauce to a boil. After that, cook, covered, for three to five minutes on low heat. Add arrowroot flour to the sauce and whisk it in until it gets thicker. Do not cook it for too long, or it will get too thick. Then, take it off the heat.
2. Mix cooked spaghetti squash and tuna into the sauce, then serve!

18. SAUTEED ZUCCHINI AND CARROTS

Prep Time: 10 Minutes | Cook Time: 10 Minutes

Total Time: 20 Minutes | Serving: 4

Ingredients

- 2 medium-sized carrots thinly sliced
- 1 tsp dried thyme
- 2 Tbsp clarified butter
- 2 medium-sized zucchini thinly sliced
- 1 Tbsp olive oil
- sea salt and ground black pepper

Instructions

1. Use medium-high heat to warm up a big skillet. Put the butter and oil in.
2. As soon as the cheese melts, add the carrots and zucchini. Put some
3. Salt and pepper, along with the thyme, and toss to coat.
4. Stir the vegetables every so often so they don't burn as you cook them until they are soft and lightly browned.

19. CINNAMON ROASTED SWEET POTATOES AND APPLES

Prep Time: 10 Minutes | Cook Time: 40 Minutes

Total Time: 50 Minutes | Serving: 8

Ingredients

- 1 tsp ground cinnamon
- 1 tsp sea salt
- 2 medium sweet potatoes
- 3 TBS coconut oil melted & divided
- 2 medium apples
- 2 TBS pure maple syrup

Instructions

1. Warm the oven up to 425 degrees F.
2. Set aside the large baking pan that you greased.
3. Toss cubed sweet potatoes with 2 tbsp of melted coconut oil in a large bowl. As you stir, the food will become coated.
4. Spread the sea salt out evenly by stirring it in.
5. When the oven is hot, put the sweet potatoes in and stir them around halfway through the 20 minutes. They should just start to turn brown.
6. Add the remaining tbsp of coconut oil to the apples and mix it in while the sweet potatoes are baking. Put in the cinnamon and maple syrup and mix them.
7. Put the sweet potatoes back in the oven after 20 minutes or when they start to turn brown. Then, add the apple mixture and stir everything together.
8. Put it back in the oven and bake again for 20 minutes, stirring every 10 minutes.
9. After the apples and sweet potatoes have turned brown and the maple syrup has caramelized, take them out of the oven and serve right away.

20. SWEET POTATO BROWNIES

Prep Time: 5 Minutes | Cook Time: 20 Minutes | Total Time: 25 Minutes | Serving: 6

Ingredients

- 1/2 cup of almond butter c
- 1/4 cup of cocoa powder
- 2 tbsp maple syrup
- 1/2 cup of chocolate chips Optional
- 1 cup of cooked sweet potato mashed

Instructions

1. Warm the oven up to 180C/350F, then grease a loaf pan and set them aside.
2. Put all the ingredients into a high-speed blender and blend well until you have a smooth brownie batter.
3. Place the ingredient mix in the prepared pan and bake for about 20 minutes.
4. For about five minutes, or until done. Take it out of the oven and let it cool down completely before cutting it up.

21. EGGPLANT CAPONATA

Prep Time: 8 Minutes | Cook Time: 30 Minutes | Total Time: 38 Minutes | Serving: 8

Ingredients

- 1 red bell pepper thinly sliced
- 2 onions finely diced
- 4 cups of chopped eggplants
- 2 tbsp capers
- 2 tbsp olive oil
- 3 cloves garlic
- 1/2 tsp salt
- 1/2 cup of chopped basil
- 3 tbsp white vinegar
- 4 cups of chopped tomatoes

Instructions

1. Cut up the onions and garlic and cook them in a big pan over medium heat for two to three minutes. Cut the eggplant into cubes about 1/2 inch thick and put them in the pan while it's cooking. Add salt.
2. For about 5 minutes, or until they're soft, cook the eggplant. Add more olive oil to the eggplant if it starts to look dry.
3. Put the chopped tomatoes, bell pepper, and vinegar in the pan. Let it cook over low heat for 20 minutes until the tomatoes and peppers are soft.
4. Serve with the chopped basil and capers. Have fun!

22. RAINBOW VEGGIE SALAD WITH LEMON VINAIGRETTE

Prep Time: 15 Minutes | Cook Time: 25 Minutes

Total Time: 40 Minutes | Serving: 8

Ingredients

Salad:

- 2 cups of brussels sprouts shredded
- 1 tbsp olive oil
- 2 cups of red cabbage shredded
- 3/4 cups of cashews
- 1 Tbsp olive oil
- 3 cups of chopped kale
- 2 cups of sweet potatoes diced
- 1/3 cup of dried tart cherries

Dressing:

- 1/8 tsp black pepper
- 1 tsp stone ground mustard
- 2 tsp date paste honey or maple syrup
- 1/8-1/4 tsp sea salt
- 1/3 cup of light-flavored olive oil or avocado oil
- 2 1/2 Tbsp lemon juice, about one lemon

Instructions

1. To roast the potatoes, heat the oven to 425 degrees. Add the olive oil and salt, then spread the vegetables well on a single layer on a baking sheet lined well with parchment paper for 25 minutes or until soft and brown.
2. Put the cashews on a separate baking sheet and roast them with the potatoes for the last 6 to 7 minutes or until they are toasty. If you want, you can sprinkle them with sea salt.
3. For about a minute, rub the kale with olive oil and salt until it has the texture you want. Shred the Brussels sprouts and add the cabbage, roasted cashews, cherries, and sweet potatoes.
4. For the dressing, put everything in a tall container and use an immersion blender until it's smooth. If you'd rather, you can mix the ingredients in a bowl while slowly adding the oil and whisking.
5. Mix the salad with the dressing. You can serve it right away or put it in the fridge until you're ready to serve. You can make this salad and dress it up a day ahead of time with no problems. Have fun!

23. ASIAN BRUSSEL SPROUTS

Prep Time: 10 Minutes | Cook Time: 20 Minutes

Total Time: 30 Minutes | Serving: 1

Ingredients

- 1.5 pounds Brussels sprouts trimmed
- 2 tbsp Olive Oil

Asian sauce:

- 1 ½ tbsp Mirin
- 2 tsp Honey
- ¼ cup of Water
- 3 tbsp Light Soy Sauce
- ¼ tsp Ground Ginger
- 1 tbsp Cornstarch or ¼ tsp xanthan gum
- 3 Garlic Cloves crushed
- 2 tsp Sesame Oil
- 3 tbsp Oyster Sauce

To serve:

- 1 pinch Chili Flakes
- 2 tbsp Sesame Seeds

Instructions

1. Warm the oven up to 200°C/400°F.Put parchment paper on a spacious baking sheet. Lightly oil the paper and set it aside.
2. Cut the Brussels sprouts in half and put them in a large bowl. Add olive oil and mix them around. Mix the halves to cover them evenly with oil. Throw away any outer leaves that came off the sprouts, but save them to make Brussels sprouts chips later.
3. Make sure the Brussels sprouts don't touch each other when you put them on the baking sheet. If necessary, use two baking sheets. After 15 minutes of baking and stirring, roast for another 10 to 15 minutes, until the outside is crispy and the inside is soft.
4. Sauce from Asia
5. In the meantime, put all of the above Asian sauce ingredients in a nonstick saucepan. Do not put this saucepan on the stove. As you use a whisk to mix the cornstarch into the liquids, break it up.
6. Bring it to a simmer and make it thicker over medium-high heat. Mix it every so often. If the sauce needs more sweetness, add more honey. Take it off the heat.
7. Toast the Brussels sprouts and then put them in a serving dish. Pour the warm, sticky sauce over the sprouts.
8. Add sesame seeds and a pinch of chili flakes before serving after stirring to combine.
9.

24. CROCKPOT BBQ BEEF

Prep Time: 20 Minutes | Cook Time: 8 Hours

Total Time: 8 Hours 20 Minutes | Serving: 8

Ingredients

- 4pound chuck roast
- 2 tbsp ghee (or coconut oil for dairy-free)

- 1 onion, diced
- Sea salt and pepper

For the sauce:

- 1 cup of coconut aminos
- 1/2 cup of tomato paste
- 1/4 cup of white vinegar
- 2 tbsp mustard

- 1 tbsp garlic powder
- 1 tbsp onion powder
- 1 tbsp chili powder
- 1 tbsp smoked paprika

Instructions

1. Cut the roast into four pieces, and sprinkle a little salt and pepper on each one. Cut the onion up the way it says to and put it in the slow cooker.
2. To make the BBQ sauce, put all of the sauce's ingredients in a bowl and mix them well with a whisk. For later use, put half of the sauce in a container and put it in the fridge.
3. Bring a big pan to medium heat and add Ghee. When it's hot, add the roast pieces and sear them on each side for four to five minutes. After searing the first two sides of the roast, flip it over and quickly sear the other four sides for one minute each. The shape of the roast may make it hard to sear some ends. Try your best to sear all sides.
4. In the slow cooker, put the beef on top of the onions. Add the last half of the BBQ sauce on top of everything.
5. After putting the lid on, cook on low for 8 to 10 hours.
6. If you want to shred the beef with two forks, you can do it in the slow cooker or on a cutting board. It should be well mixed with the onions and slow cooker juices or sauce. Serve with extra BBQ sauce on top if you want.

25. SLOW COOKER BEEF STROGANOFF

Prep Time: 5 Minutes | Cook Time: 6 Hours

Total Time: 6 Hours 5 Minutes | Serving: 6

Ingredients

- 1/4 cup of coconut aminos
- 1.5 lbs sirloin steak tips
- 3 cloves garlic minced
- 1 1/4 cup of beef broth
- 1/2 large white onion chopped
- 1/2 cup of canned coconut milk
- 10ounce sliced mushrooms

- 3 tbsp arrowroot starch***
- Salt and pepper to taste
- 1/4 cup of red wine vinegar
- 1/2 tsp garlic powder
- 2 tbsp water
- 1/2 tsp onion powder

Instructions

1. Put the beef in the slow cooker, and then add the mushrooms, onions, and garlic on top of it.
2. Put the broth, soy sauce, vinegar, onion powder, and garlic powder in a different bowl and mix them. Add to the beef and vegetables.
3. Make sure the heat is low, and let it cook for 5 hours.
4. After five hours, add the coconut cream.
5. Add arrowroot starch and water to a different small bowl and mix them. Add to the crock pot.
6. Let it cook for another 30 minutes to an hour or until the beef is soft and the sauce gets thick.
7. Serve it with rice or cauliflower rice.
8. For Instant Pot: Press the sauté button on your Instant Pot. Add about a tab of olive or avocado oil to the pan's bottom once it's hot. To make garlic, add it after the onions and cook for another minute or two. Click on "cancel."
9. Add garlic, onion powder, and some salt and pepper to your beef. Put on top of the garlic and onion mix.
10. Put broth, coconut aminos, and vinegar in a small bowl and mix them. Put on top of the meat. Put in mushrooms.
11. Put the lid back on top of your Instant Pot. Leave it to cook for 15 minutes on high pressure. Use a natural way to let go. When you open the lid, add the cream or coconut milk and stir it in. Choose the sauté function if it needs more heat to break down.
12. Add arrowroot starch and water and mix to make it thicker.
13. Put it on top of zoodles or cauliflower rice.

26. SWEET POTATO LASAGNA (AIP)

Prep Time: Minutes | Cook Time: Minutes | Total Time:1 Hour 20 Minutes | Serving:

Ingredients

Beef:

- 1.5 TBSP olive oil
- 1 pound ground beef
- 1/2 TBSP fresh basil, chopped
- 1/2 tsp garlic powder
- 1 tsp sea salt
- 1 cup of tomato sauce

Cheese" Sauce:

- 1 TBSP extra virgin olive oil
- 1/2 tsp dried thyme
- 1/2 tsp garlic powder
- 1/2 tsp sea salt

Pinch of turmeric (optional – for yellow color):

- 1 tsp apple cider vinegar
- 1 cup of full-fat, additive-free coconut milk
- 2 TBSP tapioca starch + 1 TBSP water

Sweet Potato "Pasta

- 1 giant white-fleshed sweet potato*

Instructions

1. Set the oven to 375 F and bring a large pot of water to a boil on the stove.
2. Warm up the olive oil in a big pan over medium-low heat. Add the basil, garlic powder, salt, and ground beef. Sauté for 3 to 4 minutes, stirring now and then. After that, add the tomato sauce. Turn down the heat and cook for another 4 to 5 minutes. Take the beef off the heat and set it aside.
3. Warm up some olive oil in a small saucepan over medium-low heat to make your "cheese" sauce. It's time to bring it to a low boil. Add the turmeric (if using), apple cider vinegar, salt, and coconut milk.
4. You can make a slurry by mixing tapioca starch and water in a small bowl. When the coconut milk mixture starts to boil, add the slurry and keep whisking it until it starts to get thick. Take it off the heat and set it aside.
5. Peel your white sweet potato and cut it into slices that are at least 1/4 inch thick across the length. If you make them too thin, they won't hold together when they simmer.
6. Boil water in a large pot and add the sweet potato slices. Let them cook for two minutes. The potatoes should be just barely soft, but leave them in the water for a short time, or they will break. Take the sweet potato out of the water and set it aside.
7. In an 8-by-8-inch baking pan, put your lasagna together by starting with meat sauce, then sweet potatoes, and finally "cheese sauce." Please do it again.

8. Set the oven to 375 F and bake them for 12 to 15 minutes. Then, broil for an extra 3 to 5 minutes.

---

27. ASIAN BEEF RAMEN NOODLES

Prep Time: 7 Minutes | Cook Time: 8 Minutes | Total Time: 15 Minutes | Serving: 2

Ingredients

- 2 packets of ramen or other instant noodles
- 1 tsp oil
- 2 tsp sesame oil
- 2 garlic cloves, minced
- 1/2 onion, sliced
- 200g / 7oz beef mince
- 1 1/4 cups of (315 ml) water,
- Big handful

Sauce:

- 1 tbsp dark soy sauce
- 1 tbsp Oyster sauce
- 2 tsp Hoisin sauce
- 1 tbsp mirin

Garnishes (optional):

- Finely sliced green onion/shallots
- Sesame seeds

Instructions

1. Mix the sauce and Warm up the oils in a medium-sized pan over high heat. For one and a half minutes, until the onions become golden, add the garlic and onion.
2. When you add the beef, break it up as you cook it until it goes from pink to light brown.
3. After you add the sauce, cook for two to three minutes or until the sugars are well caramelized
4. Move the beef to the side so that the noodles have room. Put noodles in water after you add water.
5. It would help if you waited 45 seconds and then turn.
6. Wait thirty seconds, then separate the noodles, and then mix them with the beef.
7. Mix in the bean sprouts and cook the noodles for one minute or until the sauce thins out enough to coat them.
8. Put the green onions and sesame seeds on the top and serve right away.

28. SLOW-COOKED ASIAN POT ROAST

Prep Time: 10 Minutes | Cook Time: Minutes

Total Time: 4 Hours 10 Minutes | Serving: 8

Ingredients

- Add Hy-Vee salt
- Hy-Vee salt
- Hy-Vee ground black pepper
- 2 (1-lbs.) pkgs. Hy-Vee Short
- ¼ c. hoisin sauce
- 3 lbs. Hy-Vee Angus Reserve beef
- 2 c. Hy-Vee no-salt-added beef broth
- Add Hy-Vee no-salt-added beef broth
- Add Hy-Vee ground black pepper
- Add hoisin sauce
- Add (1-lbs.) pkgs. Hy-Vee Short

Instructions

1. Put salt and pepper on the beef all over. Fill a 4-quart slow cooker with the food. Put hoisin sauce and beef broth in the slow cooker. Put the lid on top and set the temperature to LOW for 4 hours or HIGH for 2 hours.
2. Put Short Cuts beans and vegetables in the slow cooker. Cover, and cook on LOW for another 4 hours or on HIGH for another 2 hours or until the beef reaches 165 degrees on the inside.
3. Take the beef out of the slow cooker and use two forks to shred it. Strain the vegetables from the broth. If you want, you can save the broth. Add the reserved broth to the sliced beef if you're going to. Serve right away.

29. PALEO & WHOLE30 KOREAN SLOPPY JOES

Prep Time: 2 Minutes | Cook Time: 20 Minutes

Total Time: 22 Minutes | Serving: 6

Ingredients

- 1 tbsp avocado oil
- 2pound lean ground beef
- 1 medium onion diced
- 4 garlic cloves minced
- 1/2 inch ginger minced
- 2 tsp arrowroot starch
- 2 green onions sliced for garnish
- Sesame seeds for garnish

Sauce:

- 1/4 pear cored and roughly chopped (or use 1/2 if you like sweeter sloppy joes)
- 3/4 cup of coconut aminos
- 1/2 cup of bone broth
- 2 tbsp sugar-free ketchup or sub with gochujang
- 2 tbsp rice wine vinegar
- 2 tbsp toasted sesame oil
- 1/2 tsp sea salt
- 1/2 tsp ground black pepper
- Optional: 1/2 tsp Korean red pepper flakes or red pepper flakes

Instructions

1. Blend all sauce ingredients until combined. Remove from the table:

Instant Pot Method:

1. Start the Instant Pot and press Saute. When "Hot," add avocado oil.
2. Add ground beef and onion and break it up until it is no longer pink, 6-7 minutes.
3. Put some garlic and ginger and sauté for 1 minute more.
4. After pressing Cancel, use an oven mitt to remove the pot to drain fat carefully. I poured it over a colander and returned the meat to the bank.
5. Restart the Instant Pot and add the sauce.
6. Close the lid and set the pressure valve to seal. Heat on HIGH for 6 minutes.
7. Let it release pressure for 10 minutes before opening the lid after it beeps.
8. Then, return the Instant Pot to Saute and add arrowroot starch.
9. Remove from heat after 5 more minutes of simmering and thickening. Salt as needed after tasting.
10. Before serving, add green onions and sesame seeds.

Stove-top method:

1. Heat avocado oil in a skillet (large) on medium.
2. Add ground beef and onion and break it up until it is no longer pink, 6-7 minutes.
3. Sauté for another minute after adding ginger and garlic.
4. Fat should drain into the sink over a colander.
5. Add sauce and mix well. Keep stirring for 6-7 minutes to reduce the sauce.
6. If too much liquid remains, add arrowroot starch and simmer for 5 minutes to thicken.
7. Salt as needed after tasting.
8. Before serving, add green onions and sesame seeds.

30. CHICKEN RANCH PALEO WHOLE30 STUFFED PEPPERS

Prep Time: 15 Minutes | Cook Time: 30 Minutes | Total Time: 45 Minutes | Serving: 4

Ingredients

Peppers:

- 4-5 assorted bell peppers remove seeds and stems
- 2-3 cups of cauliflower rice
- 2-3 cups of cooked shredded chicken breast

Sauce:

- 1 cup of fresh parsley
- 1 cup of fresh cilantro
- 1/2 cup of olive oil
- lime juice from 1 lime
- 1-2 garlic cloves
- 1 jalapeño pepper remove stem
- 1/2 tsp salt

Ranch:

- 1/4 cup of paleo mayonnaise
- 1/4 cup of full-fat coconut milk
- 1 garlic cloves
- 1/4 cup of fresh parsley
- 1 tbsp fresh dill
- lemon juice from 1/2 lemon
- 1/4 tsp sea salt

Instructions

1. Preheat oven to 350F.
2. Smoothen sauce ingredients in a food processor or blender.
3. Smoothen ranch dressing ingredients in a food processor or blender.
4. Remove bell pepper tops and seeds. Put peppers in a casserole.
5. Mix cauliflower rice, shredded chicken, and sauce in a bowl. Fill peppers with this mixture.
6. Bake peppers 50 minutes at 350F. Then add ranch dressing

31. PALEO TURKEY BURGERS WITH SPINACH – LOW FODMAP

Prep Time: 15 Minutes | Cook Time: 30 Minutes

Total Time: 45 Minutes | Serving: 4

Ingredients

- 1 pound ground turkey, aim for at least 7% fat
- 1 tsp ground black pepper
- 3/4 tsp sea salt
- 2 spring onions, chopped - use the green parts only for Low FODMAP
- 1 cup of spinach, chopped - measure after chopping
- 1 tbsp coconut aminos, can sub with tamari
- 1 egg
- 1/4 cup of tapioca flour
- oil for frying

Instructions

1. Put the ground turkey, salt, pepper, spring onions, spinach, coconut aminos, and egg in a large bowl. Mix the ingredients.
2. Do not beat the tapioca flour in.
3. Split the meat into four pieces. Shape into round patties that are about 2 inches thick and 4 inches wide.
4. Get the oil hot in a pan. To cook the patties thoroughly, add them to the hot oil and cook for 20 seconds per side. It should be 165°F on the inside.
5. Please put it in lettuce wraps and top with sliced tomatoes, onion, or anything else you like. To make it low FODMAP, don't add tomato or onion.

32. KETO BEEF ENCHILADAS

Prep Time: 25 Minutes | Cook Time: 20 Minutes

Total Time: 45 Minutes | Serving: 4

Ingredients

- 1 medium yellow onion, chopped
- 1 pound ground beef
- 1 tbsp avocado oil
- 1 batch of homemade keto red enchilada sauce
- 10-ounce bag of frozen cauliflower rice
- keto-friendly wraps
- 1 cup of Mexican blend shredded cheese
- Toppings: fresh cilantro, avocado, sour cream, jalapeno, olives, and other toppings
- 1 tsp kosher salt

Instructions

1. Set the rack in the mid position of the oven and heat it to 350oF.
2. On medium heat, warm up your cast iron pan. To the hot pan, add the onion, ground beef, avocado oil, and salt. It will take about 5 to 10 minutes of cooking, stirring the meat now and then until it's almost done and the onions are soft.
3. Add the frozen cauliflower rice to the ground beef and keep cooking for another 5 minutes or until the cauliflower rice is fully thawed and the water is gone. The ground beef's flavor will soak into the cauliflower rice, making the meat last longer for less money. In addition, it adds more vegetables to the dish—one of my absolute favorite tricks.
4. Finally, add 1/4 cup of the enchilada sauce to the ground beef mix and mix it well. Please turn off the heat and mix it all.
5. Put together the enchiladas. Distribute approximately 1/4 cup of the enchilada sauce evenly across the base of your 9x13 baking dish. Layer a quarter cup of the ground beef mixture onto an assembled wrap. Sprinkle with 1 tbsp of shredded cheese. It would help if you rolled it up like a cigar and put it in the baking dish. Do the same thing with the rest of the wraps until the baking dish is entire.
6. Place a layer of shredded cheese on top and add about 1/2 cup of enchilada sauce (or more if you like).
7. Put the enchiladas in the oven with the lid off for 20 to 25 minutes or until they are warm and the cheese melts.
8. Serve warm with any toppings you want.
9. Refrigerated leftovers will last at least 5 days in an airtight container, or freeze them for at least 6 months.

33. GROUND BEEF CURRY / PAKISTANI KEEMA CURRY

Prep Time: 10 Minutes | Cook Time: 35 Minutes | Total Time: 45 Minutes | Serving: 6

Ingredients

- 3 medium potatoes
- 1/8 tsp ginger
- 1/8 tsp turmeric
- 2 1/2 – 3 cups of peas
- 2 1/4 tsp salt
- 1/8 tsp cinnamon
- 1/8 tsp pepper

- 2 1/2 – 3 cups of tomatoes
- 1 cup of chopped onion
- 1 clove garlic (minced)
- 2 – 3 tbsp oil
- 1 1/2 tbsp curry powder
- 1 pound ground beef

Instructions

In a big pan, melt butter or oil.

1. Add the garlic and onion. If you're using minced garlic, add a little water to make it liquid again.
2. Observe because garlic burns quickly as it cooks until the onion softens and the garlic starts to brown.
3. Cook the meat all the way through.
4. Put in the spices, salt, and curry. Mix well.
5. Cut up the potatoes.
6. Put tomatoes and potatoes in the pan. Bring the water to a slow boil. Turn down the heat, cover, and cook for another 10 to 15 minutes or until the potatoes are done.
7. Place the peas in the pan and cook them until they are completely soft.
8. You can eat it by itself or with rice or cauliflower.

For the Instant Pot:

1. In a pan, melt butter or oil.
2. After putting butter in the Instant Pot, add the onion, garlic, and meat. If you used minced garlic, you may need to add a little water to make it liquid again.
3. Use the sauté function to cook everything well (be careful; garlic burns quickly!).
4. Put tomatoes in.
5. Put in the spices, salt, and curry.
6. Put potatoes in.
7. Put the pressure on high for 0 minutes and cook. After 5 minutes, quickly let the stress out.
8. Add the frozen peas.
9. Set the timer for 0 minutes and cook it again under high pressure. Quickly let the stress go out.

34. EASY CURRY BEEF BOWLS RECIPE

Prep Time: 5 Minutes | Cook Time: 15 Minutes

Total Time: 20 Minutes | Serving: 4

Ingredients

For the beef:

- 3 tbsp Soy Sauce
- ¼ cup of Water
- 2 tsp Sesame Oil
- 1 ½ tbsp Mirin
- 3 Garlic Cloves crushed
- ¼ tsp Ground Ginger
- 2 tsp Honey
- 1 tbsp Cornstarch or ¼ tsp xanthan gum
- 3 tbsp Oyster Sauce

For the rest of the bowls:

1. 4 cups of greens
2. Parsley, chopped (for garnish)
3. 2 cups of cauliflower rice or white rice

Instructions

1. In a small bowl, mix the spices and set them aside. Chop the shallot.
2. Set a big pan on medium heat and add the coconut oil. Insert the beef and shallot after the cheese has melted. It should take about 6-7 minutes of cooking without breaking up the meat.
3. Add the seasoning and mix it all. After that, stir in the tomato paste for one minute.
4. With the heat turned down to medium-low, add the coconut milk and quickly bring to a simmer. Cover and cook for three to four minutes or until the beef is fully cooked.
5. While the beef is cooking, put together the bowls. Add cauliflower or white rice to a bed of greens to start. Add the beef mixture on top, and then sprinkle chopped parsley on top. Have fun!

35. SHEET PAN CHICKEN AND VEGGIES

Prep Time: 15 Minutes | Cook Time: 35 Minutes

Total Time: 50 Minutes | Serving: 4

Ingredients

- 2 tsp fresh thyme
- ½ tsp fine salt
- ½ tbsp olive oil or avocado oil
- 12ounce baby red potatoes
- ½ tsp black pepper
- 3–4 garlic cloves, minced
- 12ounce green beans
- 1 tbsp fresh rosemary
- 1½–2 lbs. bone-in, skin-on chicken thighs
- 12ounce whole carrots
- 1 medium red onion, cut into wedges

Instructions

1. Warm the oven up to 425ºF. Put parchment paper around the edges of a large baking sheet with a rim.
2. Put the chopped herbs and vegetables right on the baking sheet and toss them with oil.
3. On top of the vegetables, put the chicken thighs.
4. Add some salt and pepper to the chicken and vegetables.
5. Three to five minutes at medium heat should be enough to cook the chicken through and make the baby potatoes soft. Turn and toss the vegetables a few times while they're cooking.

36. KETO INSTANT POT THAI SHRIMP SOUP

Prep Time: 6 Minutes | Cook Time: 5 Minutes

Total Time: 18 Minutes | Serving: 6

Ingredients

- 1 tbsp coconut aminos paleo whole30
- 2 tbsp fish sauce
- 2 cloves garlic minced
- 1 tbsp grated fresh ginger root
- ½ tsp freshly ground black pepper
- 1 13.66-ounce can of unsweetened, full-fat coconut milk
- ½ pound 225g medium shrimp
- 4 cups of chicken broth
- 3 tbsp chopped fresh cilantro
- ½ yellow onion diced
- 1 stalk lemongrass bruised and finely chopped
- 1 tsp sea salt
- 1 cup of sliced fresh white mushrooms
- 2 tbsp fresh lime juice
- 2½ tsp red curry paste
- 2 tbsp unsalted butter or Ghee divided in half

Instructions

1. Once, press the Sauté button. Add 1 tbsp of butter once the inner pot is hot. When the butter melts well, add the shrimp and stir them around until they turn pink and start to curl. Move the shrimp right away to a medium-sized bowl. Put away.
2. Add the last tbsp of butter to the inside of the pot. When the butter melts, put some onions and garlic. Sauté until the onions become clear and the garlic smells good. To turn off the heat, press "Cancel."
3. Spice it up with lemongrass, mushrooms, fish sauce, coconut aminos or tamari sauce, lime juice, black pepper, sea salt, and grated ginger root. Use a stir to mix.
4. Cover, lock the lid, and turn the handle that lets steam out to the "Sealing" position. Pick-Up Pressure: Set the timer for 5 minutes and cook on High. Once the cooking time is up, release the rest of the pressure by flipping the steam release handle to "Venting" and leaving the pot alone for 5 minutes. To turn off the heat, press "Cancel."
5. Take off the lid. Stir the shrimp and coconut milk into the pot.
6. The "more or high" setting will light up when you press the Sauté button twice. Now, let the soup boil. Press "Cancel" to turn off the heat once it starts to boil. Give the soup two minutes to cool down in the pot.
7. Put the soup into bowls, top with cilantro for decoration, and serve.

37. EASIEST SALSA VERDE CHICKEN

Prep Time: 5 Minutes | Cook Time: 2 Hours

Total Time: 2 Hour 5 Minutes | Serving: 6

Ingredients

- 16ounce roasted salsa verde, **check labels for Whole 30 compliance
- salt, to taste
- 1 1/2 lbs raw skinless chicken tenders or chicken breast
- 1/8 tsp ground cumin
- 1/4 tsp garlic powder
- 1/8 tsp oregano

Instructions

1. Cover the chicken with oregano, cumin, garlic powder, and salt. Keep the chicken in the bottom of the slow cooker.
2. Put the lid on and cook on HIGH for two hours or low for four hours.

38. INSTANT POT CHICKEN TORTILLA-LESS SOUP

Prep Time: 5 Minutes | Cook Time: 20 Minutes

Total Time: 45 Minutes | Serving: 4

Ingredients

- 2 tsp chili powder
- 1 medium onion chopped
- For the Soup
- 1 14-ounce can full-fat coconut milk
- 1 tsp cumin
- 2 boneless chicken breasts
- 1 14.5-ounce can of chicken broth
- 1 ½ tsp salt
- 1 tsp smoked paprika
- 2 10-ounce cans of tomatoes
- 1 tsp dried oregano
- 1 tsp onion powder
- 1-3 tsp chipotle pepper powder
- 2 zucchinis chopped or cut into ½-inch half moons
- 2 tsp garlic powder

Instructions

1. Salt chicken breasts that don't have any bones or skin on them. Keep the chicken breasts in the Instant Pot. Add the rest of the ingredients one by one, starting with the zucchini.
2. Put the lid back on the pot. Twelve hours of high-pressure cooking. After ten minutes of letting the pressure drop on its own, use the manual release. Take the chicken breasts out of the pan and add the coconut milk. Put the Instant Pot into Sauté mode and stir everything together.
3. Cut the chicken into small pieces or shred it, then add it back to the soup. When you serve it hot, you can add any toppings you like.

39. HEALTHY SESAME CHICKEN CHOPPED SALAD

Prep Time: 15 Minutes | Cook Time: 15 Minutes

Total Time: 30 Minutes | Serving: 6

Ingredients

For the Dressing:

- 3 tbsp avocado oil
- 1/4 cup of red wine vinegar (or apple cider vinegar)
- 1/3 cup of coconut aminos
- 1 tsp onion powder
- 2 tbsp toasted sesame oil
- 2 tbsp minced ginger
- 1 tsp salt
- 1/2 tsp pepper

For the Salad:

- 2 cups of shredded or matchstick carrots
- 4 diced green onions
- 1.5 pounds boneless, skinless chicken thighs
- 1 can Mandarin oranges
- 1/2 red cabbage, thinly sliced
- 1 tbsp black sesame seeds
- 1/2 large green cabbage, thinly sliced
- 1/2 cup of packed cilantro
- 1 tbsp white sesame seeds
- 1 cup of sliced almonds

Instructions

1. In a bowl, mix together all of the dressing's ingredients.
2. Put the chicken and about 3–4 tbsp of dressing in a plastic bag. Let it sit for at least 30 minutes.
3. In a spacious skillet over medium-low heat, cook the chicken for 6 to 8 minutes on each side or until fully cooked. Alternatively, you can grill the chicken.
4. Let it cool to room temperature before cutting it up and putting it in the salad.
5. In a spacious bowl, mix all the salad ingredients except the dressing and chicken.
6. Add the chicken to the salad when it's cool.
7. Add the dressing and mix it well.

40. PALEO SALMON CAKES

Prep Time: 10 Minutes | Cook Time: 8 Minutes | Total Time: 38 Minutes | Serving: 6

Ingredients

- 1/3 cup of finely chopped parsley, packed
- 1/2 Tbsp kosher salt
- 2 large eggs
- 2/3 cup of almond meal
- 1/2 tsp freshly ground black pepper
- 1 large sweet potato
- 2 14.75-ounce cans of Wild Alaskan Salmon
- 1 tsp ground cumin
- 1 Tbsp hot sauce
- 2 Tbsp finely chopped onion
- 1.25 tsp paprika sweet OR smoked
- 1 Tbsp freshly squeezed lemon juice
- 2 Tbsp organic coconut oil

Instructions

1. Clean sweet potato and make several fork-holes. Microwave until soft on a paper towel-wrapped plate. My microwave has "potato" mode. I think it takes 8–9 minutes, but check every couple of days to avoid overcooking.
2. If you choose not to use the microwave, you can bake or pressure cook the potato and store it in the fridge for a few days, mashed and ready.
3. After cooling for a few minutes, remove potato flesh from the skin and mash it with a fork to remove lumps. Mix in a large bowl.
4. Almond meal, chopped parsley, onion, lemon juice, hot sauce, salt, cumin, paprika, black pepper, and eggs.
5. Open wild salmon cans and drain most of the liquid. I used Trader Joe's canned skin-and-bone Wild Pink Alaskan Salmon.
6. Find the "split," where two or more salmon pieces are pushed together into the can by holding the canned salmon. Salmon naturally separate here, and most of the skin and bones are here. Gently scrape or mix the skin and bones off with your hands.
7. If more "splits" appear, separate the salmon again and repeat. Last, crush the canned salmon into the mixing bowl with your fingers.
8. Mix well. Line a fridge-sized baking sheet or plate with parchment paper.
9. With a 1/3 measuring cup, scoop evenly sized salmon cakes (flattened bottoms) to make 12 patties (sometimes 13 or 14).
10. Chill in the fridge for 20 minutes or all day (freeze any not cooked within 12–24 hours).
11. To cook:
12. Cook six patties in a large frying pan with mid-range heat. When hot, add 1 tbsp of coconut oil or Ghee per six patties.
13. Melt fat completely and heat it.
14. Add patties and cook for 4 minutes.
15. Turn gently and cook for 4 more minutes.
16. Serve hot and enjoy!

41. CREAMY CARROT AND GINGER SOUP (DAIRY-FREE)

Prep Time: 5 Minutes | Cook Time: 30 Minutes

Total Time: 35 Minutes | Serving: 5

Ingredients

- 1 clove garlic minced
- 1 14ounce can of coconut cream
- 1 tbsp coconut oil
- 1/2 tsp salt + more to taste
- 24-32ounce vegetable broth**
- 1pound carrots peeled and chopped
- 3 tbsp chopped fresh ginger*
- 1 medium-sized yellow onion chopped

Instructions

For the Stovetop:

1. Start by heating a spacious skillet on medium-high. Melt coconut oil.
2. Stir in onion, garlic, and ginger. Cook onion until fragrant and almost clear, 5 minutes.
3. Boil carrots and vegetable stock.
4. Reduce heat to simmer. Cook carrots for 25 minutes until soft. Stir in coconut milk or cream slowly.
5. Smoothen soup with an immersion blender. Blend in batches with a regular blender. Salt to taste. Serve hot!

For the Instant Pot:

1. Select IP to saute. Once hot, add onion and oil. Add garlic and ginger, then saute for 2 minutes after 2-3 minutes.
2. Select IP cancel. Add 3 cups of (24ounce) broth and carrots. Safeguard the lid. Choose manual and cook on high pressure for 6 minutes.
3. Release quickly. Add coconut milk and salt (to taste).
4. Blend until creamy with a blender or immersion blender.
5. Serve hot!

42. PALEO CHICKEN AND BROCCOLI IN THE INSTANT POT

Prep Time: 10 Minutes | Cook Time: 10 Minutes

Total Time: 20 Minutes | Serving: 2

Ingredients

- 1/4 tsp black pepper
- 1 tsp fish sauce
- 2 cloves garlic minced
- 2 tbsp arrowroot or tapioca flour
- 1/4 tsp fine sea salt
- 1/2 cup of chicken broth
- 1 "knob ginger grated or minced
- 10-12 ounces of broccoli florets
- 2 tbsp water
- 1/4 tsp apple cider vinegar
- Pinch red pepper flakes, optional
- 2 tbsp sesame oil
- 1/4 cup of coconut aminos
- Sesame seeds for garnish
- 1pound boneless skinless chicken breasts

Instructions

1. In the Instant Pot, combine chicken, broth, coconut aminos, sesame oil, fish sauce, ginger, garlic, salt, and pepper. Cover and cook for 8 minutes on manual high pressure.
2. Once done, turn the knob for quick release.
3. Make a slurry of arrowroot and water in a small bowl. Put this in the instant pot with chicken.
4. Turn on sauté after pressing off. Stir frequently for 5 minutes to soften broccoli and reduce and thicken the sauce.
5. Mix apple cider vinegar in. Press cancel to turn it off.
6. Sprinkle sesame seeds and serve with cauliflower or white rice immediately

43. CHIPOTLE CHICKEN SALAD

Prep Time: 15 Minutes | Cook Time: 10 Minutes

Total Time: 25 Minutes | Serving: 3

Ingredients

- 1 pound chicken, cooked and diced
- 4 stalks of celery, finely chopped
- 1/4 white onion, finely chopped
- For the mayo
- ⅔ cup of avocado oil
- 1 egg
- 1 tsp lemon juice
- 1 tsp chipotle adobo sauce
- 1/4 tsp cayenne pepper
- 1/4 tsp garlic powder
- salt and pepper, to taste

Instructions

1. Combine chopped chicken, celery, and white onion.
2. Put all mayo ingredients in a tall container, put the immersion blender at the bottom, and turn it on. Keep the immersion blender on until the oil turns white and becomes mayo. It should take 30 seconds or less!
3. Mix chicken, celery, and onion with mayo.
4. Eat as you please. Fork-in lettuce. Or spoon. Anything goes with 30-second mayo and chicken salad.

44. ONE PAN THAI BASIL BEEF

Prep Time: 10 Minutes | Cook Time: 20 Minutes

Total Time: 30 Minutes | Serving: 4

Ingredients

- 1 white onion sliced
- 1 tsp kosher salt
- 1 tbsp fish sauce
- 1 pound flank steak
- 1/4 cup of cilantro
- 2 large red bell peppers julienned
- 1/3 cup of coconut aminos
- 1/4 cup of green onions
- 2 1/2 tbsp avocado oil
- 6 garlic cloves minced
- 1 tbsp arrowroot flour
- 1/4 tsp black pepper
- 1 cup of Thai basil or regular basil lightly packed & roughly chopped

Instructions

1. Cut the flank steak into thin strips that are easy to eat, and then put them in a large bowl. A twenty-minute freeze is what I like to do with my flank steak before I cut it. It helps carry out the task! Add salt, pepper, and 1/2 tbsp of avocado oil. Mix well, then set it aside.
2. For two minutes, heat a very large frying pan over medium-high heat. Put in the last two tbsp of avocado oil and heat it up for one more minute. Place the flank steak in the pan in a thin layer, being careful not to crowd it. If you need to, you can do this in two batches. For about three minutes on each side, until golden and crispy. Use tongs or a slotted spoon to take them out and put them on a big plate.
3. Put white onion and bell pepper in the pan. Stirring every now and then, cook over medium heat for about 7 minutes until the vegetables are soft all the way through. Put the steak back in the pan and cook for one minute, stirring often. Bring the coconut aminos and fish sauce to a low boil. Turn down the heat and let it simmer for three minutes or until it starts to get a little thicker. Take it off the heat and add the basil leaves.
4. Put rice in a bowl or on a plate, and then add Thai basil beef on top of it. Put green onions and fresh cilantro on top.

45. ASIAN TURKEY MEATBALLS WITH LIME SESAME DIPPING SAUCE

Prep Time: 20 Minutes | Cook Time: 15 Minutes

Total Time: 35 Minutes | Serving: 4

Ingredients

- 1/4 cup of panko crumbs
- 1-1/4 lbs 93% lean ground turkey
- 1 large egg
- 1 tbsp ginger, minced
- 1 clove ga
- garlic, minced
- 1/2 tsp kosher salt
- 1/4 cup of chopped fresh cilantro
- 3 scallions, chopped
- 1 tbsp low sodium soy sauce
- 2 tsp sesame oil

For the Dipping Sauce:

- 3 tbsp reduced-sodium soy sauce
- 1 1/2 tsp sesame oil
- 1 1/2 tbsp fresh lime juice
- 1 1/2 tbsp water
- 1 tbsp chopped fresh scallion

Instructions

1. Warm the oven up to 500°F.
2. Add the salt, scallions, garlic, ginger, cilantro, 1 tbsp of soy sauce, and 2 tbsp of sesame oil to a large bowl. Mix the ground turkey with these ingredients.
3. Mix slowly with your hands until everything is well mixed.
4. Make meatballs about the size of a quarter cup of and put them on a baking sheet.
5. About 15 to 18 minutes, or until fully cooked and browned.
6. Add the water, soy sauce, lime juice, and the last 2 tsp of oil to a bowl and mix them together.
7. Set the scallions aside after you add them.
8. Put the meatballs on a dish to serve.
9. Mix the sauce together, and then add some of it to the meatballs.
10. Put the meatballs on a plate and add the rest of the sauce to the side.

46. PALEO BUFFALO CHICKEN CASSEROLE WITH RANCH AND CAULIFLOWER RICE

Prep Time: 5 Minutes | Cook Time: 30 Minutes

Total Time: 35 Minutes | Serving: 4

Ingredients

- 4 cups of cooked chicken
- 3 cups of cauliflower rice
- 1 cup of green onions sliced

Creamy Buffalo Ranch Sauce:

- ½ cup of Whole30 mayonnaise
- ¼ cup of Whole30 ranch dressing
- ¼ cup of + 2 tbsp coconut cream
- ½ cup of hot sauce
- 1 tsp garlic p

Instructions

1. Warm the oven up to 350o F.
2. In a large bowl, mix together the chicken, cauliflower rice, and 1 cup of green onions. In a medium-sized bowl, mix all the sauce ingredients together with a whisk. Add the sauce to the chicken-rice mix and mix it well. Move to a 9x9-inch baking dish.
3. For thirty minutes, or until it bubbles. Add more ranch dressing, green onions, and chopped fresh parsley as a garnish. If you want, you can serve it with celery sticks.

47. VIETNAMESE CHICKEN PHO (PHO GA)

Prep Time: 10 Minutes | Cook Time: 60 Minutes

Total Time: 1 Hour 10 Minutes | Serving: 4

Ingredients

- 1 cinnamon stick
- 1 whole chicken
- 4 cm (1½ inch) fresh ginger,
- 8 shallots or 2 small onions
- 1 scant tbsp Maldon sea salt
- 4-star anise
- 1 tbsp fish sauce
- 1 tbsp sugar

Instructions

1. Put chicken in a big pot.
2. Add barely enough cold water to cover the chicken.
3. Start by boiling the pot, then lower the heat to medium or simmer.
4. Meanwhile, grill the shallots (or onions) and ginger on high heat until slightly charred. If you have a gas stove, you can char the vegetables over an open flame or under the oven grill.
5. Add chargrilled onions, ginger, cinnamon stick, and star anise to the pot.
6. The chicken should be tender and fall off the bones after 1–1.5 hours of simmering. The chicken size determines the cooking time.
7. Skim off impurities that rise to the surface of the stock and top up with boiling water if it has reduced significantly. I try to keep the water level constant.
8. When tender, transfer the chicken to a large bowl and let it cool before shredding.
9. Return heat to the broth after straining through a fine sieve into a clean pot.
10. Season broth with salt, sugar, and fish sauce.
11. Simmer gently for 10 minutes.
12. Taste seasoning. If the broth is too concentrated, add boiling water.
13. Put shredded chicken on top of noodles in four large bowls.
14. Pour hot broth into each bowl and add fresh herbs and toppings.

48. HONEY WALNUT SHRIMP

Prep Time: 10 Minutes | Cook Time: 10 Minutes

Total Time: 20 Minutes | Serving: 4

Ingredients

Candied walnuts:

- 2 tbsp water
- 1 tbsp unsalted butter
- 2 tbsp cane sugar
- ½ cup of walnut halves

Shrimp:

- 3 tbsp arrowroot starch
- 2 tbsp olive oil
- ½ tsp salt
- 1 pound large shrimp
- ½ tsp garlic powder

Honey Sauce:

- 2 tbsp honey
- 1 tbsp lemon juice
- 2 tbsp avocado mayonnaise

For Serving:

- Shredded green cabbage
- Rice
- Green onions

Instructions

1. Using medium-low heat, add the butter, walnuts, sugar, and water to a large nonstick skillet. As you stir, the sugar will melt and cover the walnuts. This will take about 5 minutes.
2. Put it on a piece of parchment paper right away and separate the nuts right away. Set it aside to harden, and then clean the pan.
3. To make the shrimp evenly coated, put the shrimp, arrowroot starch, garlic powder, and salt in a large bowl and stir them together.
4. While the olive oil is heating up in a large skillet over medium-high heat, add the shrimp and cook them, turning them over a few times, for about two to three minutes on each side.
5. Melt the honey and lemon juice in a small bowl and mix them together with a whisk. Put the shrimp in the sauce and toss them to mix. Place the sweet walnuts on top and
6. Put cooked shrimp on top of green cabbage shavings, sesame seeds, and green onions on a plate.

49. VIETNAMESE LEMONGRASS CHICKEN

Prep Time: 10 Minutes | Cook Time: 15 Minutes

Total Time: 1 Hour 25 Minutes | Serving: 4

Ingredients

- ¼ cup of cooking oil
- ¼ cup of rice wine vinegar (can sub apple cider vinegar)
- 2 tbsp soy sauce (gluten-free if needed)
- 2 stalks of lemongrass (inner white part only)
- 2 cloves garlic
- 2 inch piece of ginger
- 1 lime (juiced)
- 8 boneless chicken thighs
- Green onions, thinly sliced chilies, red onion, and lime (to serve)

The sriracha mayo:

- ¼ cup of mayonnaise
- 1-3 tsp sriracha (to taste)
- 1 pinch of sea salt

Instructions

1. To make the sauce smooth, put the oil, vinegar, soy sauce, garlic, ginger, lemongrass, and lime juice in a blender. Set the speed to high.
2. Cover the chicken thighs with the marinade. Put them in a shallow dish, like a baking dish. Moving the chicken thighs around a lot will cover each one with the marinade. Put the chicken in the sauce for one to two hours.
3. Make the sriracha mayo while the chicken is swimming in the sauce. In a tiny bowl, mix the mayonnaise, sriracha, and sea salt together well. Until you use it, put it in the fridge.
4. Set your grill or BBQ to medium-high heat. Take the chicken out of the marinade and throw away the marinade.
5. Put the chicken on the grill and cook it for 6 to 7 minutes on each side or until it reaches 165 degrees Fahrenheit inside.
6. Dress up the chicken after taking it off the grill and serve it with sriracha mayo on the side.

50. SWEET AND SPICY PORK LETTUCE WRAPS

Prep Time: 10 Minutes | Cook Time: 20 Minutes

Total Time: 30 Minutes | Serving: 4

Ingredients

For the sauce

- 2 tsp sriracha
- 2 tsp fresh ground ginger
- 2 cloves garlic minced
- 2 tbsp coconut aminos or soy sauce
- 1 tbsp honey omit for whole30 option
- 1 tbsp rice wine vinegar
- 2 tbsp nut butter

For the lettuce wraps:

- 1pound ground pork
- 1 (8 ounces) can of water chestnuts drained and diced
- 1 red pepper diced
- 1 cup of shredded carrots
- 1 small yellow onion diced
- Butter lettuce leaves for serving
- Topping: green onions, cilantro and crushed peanuts
- Sauce for serving (optional):
- 3 tbsp coconut aminos or soy sauce
- 1 tbsp nut butter
- 2 tsp honey
- 1 tsp sriracha

Instructions

1. Put everything for the sauce in a medium bowl and mix it together well with a whisk. Put away.
2. Put 1 tbsp of olive oil in a big pan or wok and set it over medium-high heat. Add the ground pork and cook until there is no more pink. To make it crispy, stir the pork around a few times while it's still in the hot oil. This turns the outside golden brown.
3. With the pork done, add the water chestnuts, red pepper, carrots, and onion. Put some salt and pepper on the chicken and vegetables.
4. Add the sauce and stir until it's all mixed in. For a thickening and flavor development simmer, reduce heat to medium-low and cook for around 10 minutes.
5. Take the pan off the heat and put the food in the lettuce cups. For a more substantial wrap, you should use two lettuce cups of instead of one. If you want, you can add chopped scallions, cilantro, and peanuts on top.
6. Put all the sauce ingredients in a small bowl and mix them with a whisk while the pork filling cooks. Before you serve the lettuce wraps, put sauce on top of them.

51. ORANGE CHICKEN RECIPE

Prep Time: 5 Minutes | Cook Time: 10 Minutes

Total Time: 15 Minutes | Serving: 4

Ingredients

For the Marinade:

- ½ cup of freshly squeezed orange juice
- ⅓ cup of Asian seasoned rice vinegar
- 1/4 cup of regular soy sauce
- zest of one orange
- 1 tsp ground ginger
- 1 cup of chicken broth
- ½ cup of white sugar
- 2 TB Sriracha, depending on the desired heat level
- 2 TB cornstarch
- 4 cloves garlic, finely minced

For the Chicken:

- 2 large eggs
- Optional: sesame seeds and green onions
- 1pound boneless, skinless chicken breasts
- 1 cup of cornstarch in a pie pan
- 1 cup of peanut oil for frying

Instructions

1. Make the Marinade: Put all the ingredients for the marinade in a bowl and whisk them together well. Mix the chicken with 1/2 cup of the marinade, making sure that the marinade covers all of the chicken pieces. Soak it in the sauce for at least 30 minutes.
2. Boil and Thicken: In the meantime, heat the remaining marinade in a medium saucepan over medium-low heat and stir it around a lot. When the sauce boils, it will get thicker. Turn off the heat when the sauce is well thick. While you fry the chicken, keep the sauce warm.
3. Coat: Take the chicken out of the marinade and throw away any extra sauce. Gently dip a few chicken pieces at a time into the egg mixture in the pan. Let the extra eggs drip off, and then coat the chicken pieces in the cornstarch in the pan. Press to cover well. To cover all the details, do it again and again.
4. To fry, put oil in a large saucepan and heat it over medium-high to high heat until it's boiling. It will take about one to two minutes to cook after adding the chicken pieces. Be careful not to crowd the pan. Working in groups, fry the chicken and then put it on paper towels.
5. Toss and Serve: Put the chicken and warm sauce together, and then serve right away. Serve with rice and any toppings you like.

52. TRADER JOE'S POTSTICKER STIR-FRY

Prep Time: 5 Minutes | Cook Time: 15 Minutes

Total Time: 20 Minutes | Serving: 4

Ingredients

- Kosher salt and freshly ground black pepper
- 1 (16-ounce) bag of frozen Trader
- 1 (16-ounce) bag of frozen Trader
- 1 cup of Trader Dipping Sauce

Instructions

1. Put 2 tbsp of olive oil in a spacious skillet and set it over medium-high heat. Toss in the veggies and add the pepper and salt—Stir-fry for around 5 minutes or until the vegetables are almost soft.
2. Place the potstickers in a single layer, pleat-side up, in the space to the side. Fry for three minutes. Cover, add a little water, and steam for three minutes.
3. Toss everything in the gyoza sauce to cover it, then serve.

53. KETO WONTON-LESS SOUP - PALEO, WHOLE30

Prep Time: 35 Minutes | Cook Time: 25 Minutes | Total Time: 50 Minutes | Serving: 10

Ingredients

For the meatballs:

- 1 ½ pounds ground pork
- 3 tbsp coconut aminos
- 2 tbsp and more 1 tsp toasted sesame oil, divided
- 1 tsp gluten-free oyster sauce
- 1 tsp fish sauce
- 1 tsp grated fresh ginger
- ¼ tsp crushed red pepper flakes
- 2 cloves garlic, minced
- 2 green onions, chopped
- 1 large pastured egg

For the broth:

- 8 cups of chicken stock
- 2 cups of water
- 2 tsp of oyster sauce
- 1/2 cup of gluten-free soy sauce or coconut aminos
- 2 big spoonfuls of fish sauce
- 2 tsp of fresh ginger grate
- ½ tsp of red pepper flakes, broken up
- 5 large cremini mushrooms, cut very thinly
- 1 bunch of thinly sliced green onions 14-ounce bag of coleslaw mix

Instructions

1. Put oyster sauce, fish sauce, ginger, red pepper flakes, garlic, green onions, egg, coconut aminos, and 1 tsp of sesame oil in a spacious bowl. Mix until everything is well combined. Make meatballs that are about the size of a pea. About 40 meatballs should come out of it.
2. Put the last 2 tbsp of sesame oil in a stock pot and heat it over medium-high heat. Put the meatballs in the bank. Turn the meatballs over and cook them all the way through. Add some chicken stock to the pool if they start to stick. Take the meatballs out of the pot and set them aside.
3. Add water, oyster sauce, ginger, fish sauce, coconut aminos, and red pepper flakes to the pot. Once it starts to boil, turn down the heat and let it simmer. Let it cook for 10 minutes.
4. Combine the cabbage, mushrooms, and meatballs in the broth. Let it cook for five more minutes before serving.

54. PALEO CHICK-FIL-A CHICKEN

Prep Time: Minutes | Cook Time: 15 Minutes

Total Time: 15 Minutes | Serving:

Ingredients

- coconut or avocado oil to cook in
- 2 chicken breasts
- 1/2 tsp garlic powder
- 1 egg*
- 1/2 cup of pickle juice*
- 1/4 cup of tapioca or arrowroot flour
- 3/4 tsp paprika
- 1/3 cup of almond flour*
- 1/4 tsp pepper
- 1 tsp salt
- 1/4 tsp onion powder

Instructions

1. Mix pickle juice and cut the chicken breast in a bowl. Cover well and put in a fridge for 30 minutes overnight. Longer marinating intensifies the pickle flavor.
2. Remove marinated meat from the fridge. Strain the chicken to remove pickle juice. Use a paper towel or a rag that can be used again to dry the chicken. Avoid skipping this drying step to keep breading on chicken!
3. Crack and scramble egg in a small bowl. Stir egg and chicken pieces in a medium bowl until coated. To remove excess egg from the chicken, strain again. Shake the filter several times to remove excess. The breading sticks better to chicken if you withdraw more lots.
4. In a small size bowl, mix almond flour with pepper. Sprinkle over drained chicken in a medium bowl. Stir gently to coat all pieces in breading.
5. Heating oil in a medium saucepan on medium-high. I use 1/4" oil. Put chicken pieces in the oil when it's hot. Leave space between elements in the pan.
6. Cook each side for 5-6 minutes until crispy golden brown. Repeat until pieces are dry and pink-free.
7. Airfry chicken at 350 for 10 minutes, flipping halfway.
8. These are great frozen chicken nugget substitutes. Cook as directed above, then freeze in a single layer on a cooling rack. After freezing, store in a sealed container for 3+ months. Reheat in the microwave, oven at 400 for 10 minutes, or air fryer at 350 for 5-7 minutes.
9. Want fresh cooking? You could prep and freeze these raw (following instructions until marinated and breaded) and cook on the stove or air fryer from the freezer with the above recipe, adding a few minutes.

55. SPINACH ARTICHOKE DIP

Prep Time: 5 Minutes | Cook Time: 25 Minutes

Total Time: 30 Minutes | Serving: 8

Ingredients

- 2 tsp Olive oil
- 4ounce Spinach
- 4ounce Cream cheese
- 2 tbsp Mayonnaise
- 2 tbsp Sour cream
- One (14.5ounce) can of artichoke hearts in water
- 1/4 cup of Grated parmesan cheese
- 4 cloves Garlic
- 1/4 tsp Black pepper
- 2/3 cup of Mozzarella cheese

Instructions

1. Set the oil on medium heat in a medium-sized pan. Put in the spinach. Stir the spinach every once in a while for two to three minutes or until it is wilted and bright green. You can microwave the spinach for about two to three minutes. Leave to cool. Putting the bowl into a giant bowl with ice can speed up the cooling process, but it's not necessary.
2. Heat the oven to 350 degrees F (177 degrees C) while the spinach cools.
3. While that's going on, heat the cream cheese in the microwave or over low heat in a medium saucepan. Add the mayonnaise, grated Parmesan cheese, chopped artichoke hearts, sour cream, minced garlic, black pepper, and half of the shredded mozzarella once the cheese has melted enough to stir. Use a stir to mix.
4. Once it's cool enough to touch, roll the spinach into a ball and squeeze it a few times to get rid of as much water as you can. Mix the spinach with the artichokes.
5. Move the dip to a large ramekin or a small ceramic appetizer dish. Use a spatula to make the top smooth. Add the rest of the shredded mozzarella on top.
6. If you want it hot and bubbly, bake it for 20 to 30 minutes. Warm up and serve.

56. AHI TUNA POKE BOWL

Prep Time: 45 Minutes | Cook Time: 30 Minutes

Total Time: 1 Hour 15 Minutes | Serving: 6

Ingredients

Ahi Tuna:

- 1.5 lbs. Ahi Tuna Steaks 2 1.5-inch steaks
- 1/3 cup of soy sauce
- 1 tsp red chili sauce
- 1 tsp fresh grated ginger
- 1 tbsp lime juice
- 4 tbsp sesame seeds
- 4 tbsp olive oil

Cilantro White Rice:

- 1 cup of long-grain white rice
- 1.5 cups of water*
- 1/4 cup of chopped fresh cilantro

Salad:

- I cup of sliced cucumbers
- 1 cup of sliced radishes
- 1 cup of sliced cabbage
- 2 tbsp apple cider vinegar
- 2 tbsp lime juice
- 1/4 tsp salt

Poke Bowl Dressing:

- 3 tbsp drippy almond butter
- 1 tsp sriracha
- 1 tbsp soy sauce
- 1 tbsp water
- 1 tbsp lime juice

Poke Bowl:

- 2 large avocados halved and sliced
- Sesame seeds to taste

Instructions

Ahi Tuna:

1. Begin by transferring the tuna steaks to a sizable basin or a plastic bag.
2. Combine lime juice, grated ginger, soy sauce, chili sauce, and ahi tuna in a small mason jar for a delicious marinade. Reduce the elasticity of the After adding all of the ingredients to the pot, shake it to combine. Disperse the mixture evenly over the ahi tuna steaks.
3. Seal the plastic bag. The steaks will benefit from marinating for at least half an hour in the refrigerator, preferably more time.

4. Take the ahi tuna steaks out of the marinade after taking them out of the fridge. After you pour the sesame seeds onto a plate, coat both tuna steaks thoroughly—steaks including sesame seeds.
5. Put 2 tbsp of olive Saute the oil in a big skillet over medium-high heat. Sear one tuna steak for 30 seconds to 2 minutes per side once the olive oil begins to smell good.*
6. Turn the tuna steaks over for the second time.
7. After searing tuna steaks, set aside to rest for 2 minutes before slicing thinly.

Cilantro White Rice:

1. Place white rice and water into a medium saucepan. Turn the heat to high and bring it to a boil.
2. Once boiling, reduce heat to low and cover. Let simmer for around 15 minutes or until all water has absorbed.
3. Remove from heat and let cool for 10 minutes. Add cilantro and mix.
4. Set aside for later.

The salad:

1. In a big bowl, combine all of the salad ingredients and toss to combine.
2. Save for a subsequent time.

Dressing for Poke Bowls:

1. Transfer the dressing ingredients to an individual mason jar.
2. Combine all ingredients by shaking vigorously.
3. Save for a subsequent time.

Seafood Bowls:

1. Four poke bowls can be made now! Spread half a cup of cooked white rice evenly across all of the serving dishes.
2. Split the seared tuna in half and top each bowl with a quarter of the salad.
3. Top each bowl with a quarter of an avocado and top with the almond butter dressing.
4. Add a final touch by dusting with sesame seeds.

57. PALEO SESAME CHICKEN {WHOLE30}

Prep Time: 15 Minutes | Cook Time: 20 Minutes

Total Time: 35 Minutes | Serving: 6

Ingredients

Sesame sauce:

- 2/3 cup of water warmed slightly
- 3 Tbsp rice vinegar
- 2 tsp arrowroot flour or tapioca
- 1 Tbsp sesame oil
- 1/4 cup of coconut aminos
- 1/4-1/2 tsp red pepper flakes adjust to taste
- 5 Medjool dates pitted
- 1/2 tsp garlic powder

Chicken:

- 2 pound boneless skinless chicken thighs
- 1 tsp sesame oil
- 1/2 tsp

Garlic Powder

- 1 cup of tapioca flour or arrowroot
- 1 1/4 tsp salt
- 1/4 tsp black pepper
- 2 eggs whisked
- Avocado oil or refined coconut oil

Garnish:

- 2 Tbsps sesame seeds for garnish
- Thinly sliced scallions for garnish

Instructions

Sauce:

1. Using a high-speed blender, blend all the sauce ingredients until the mixture is smooth. If necessary, scrape down the sides to add all the dates.
2. Put the sauce in a small pot and set it over medium-low heat. Stir and heat for two to three minutes until it boils. Then turn down the heat to medium-low and let it simmer. After you add the red pepper flakes, let the mixture cook for three to four more minutes until it gets a bit thicker and less watery, like a thick caramel.

Chicken:

1. Add the salt and pepper to a shallow bowl with the arrowroot or tapioca.

2. In a different, shallow bowl, beat the eggs. Pour the sesame oil over the chicken and sprinkle the garlic powder on top.
3. Using a whisk, lightly coat the chicken pieces in egg. Then, toss them in arrowroot starch and shake off the extra. Place the chicken pieces in a bowl.
4. In a big, deep, nonstick skillet, heat about 1/2 cup of oil. Once the oil is boiling, add the chicken pieces one at a time and cook them for about three minutes, turning them over until they are golden and crisp.
5. Keep the chicken on a plate lined with paper towels. Do this again with the rest of the chicken, changing the heat as needed and adding more oil if needed.
6. Bring the sesame sauce back to a low temperature and mix it with the chicken. Add green onion and sesame seeds to the top of the dish to serve. You can serve it over sautéed cauliflower rice or your favorite vegetables. Have fun!

58. GUACAMOLE DEVILED EGGS

Prep Time: 15 Minutes | Cook Time: 12 Minutes

Total Time: 27 Minutes | Serving: 12

Ingredients

- salt or garlic salt to taste
- 1 tsp fresh lemon juice
- 1-2 Tbsp mayonnaise
- 6 extra large hard-boiled eggs
- 1/2 cup of mashed avocado

Instructions

1. Cut each egg in half down the middle, and then pop the yolks out.
2. Add lemon juice to the freshly mashed avocado to keep it from turning brown.
3. In a small size bowl, mix the egg yolks, mayonnaise, and avocado. Blend with an immersion blender when the mixture is creamy and smooth. To taste, add salt or garlic salt. You can make it better by adding more lemon.
4. You can also use a small food processor to blend the ingredients, making sure to scrape down the sides as needed.
5. Put the mixture in a pastry bag with a big star tip.
6. Use a pipe to fill the egg halves that have been hollowed out.
7. Add snipped chives as a garnish.

59. EASY SAUTÉED MIXED GREENS RECIPE

Prep Time: 15 Minutes | Cook Time: 15 Minutes

Total Time: 30 Minutes | Serving: 4

Ingredients

- 1 large bunch spinach
- Sea or kosher salt, to taste
- 1 tbsp olive oil
- 1 large bunch of kale
- 2 to 3 cloves garlic, minced
- Freshly ground black pepper, to taste
- 3 large green onions, or 1 large shallot, finely chopped

Instructions

1. Get the ingredients together.
2. Run cold water over the greens and let them dry. You can also use clean towels to dry them gently.
3. Please take off the kale or chard's thicker stems and throw them away. You can leave the skinny, soft branches on. Cut it up into pieces that are bigger than bite-sized. There will be less greens after they cook down.
4. Clean the greens and put the oil in a large skillet over medium-low heat. Spread the garlic out in the oil, then sauté for another 30 seconds or until a pleasant aroma begins to emanate.
5. After you add the onions or shallot, cook for another minute or two until they become soft.
6. Add chard or kale to the pan and cook until the leaves wilt and are just barely soft. This should take about 6 to 8 minutes for chard and a little less time for kale.
7. Stir the spinach in and cook for one to two minutes, until it's just wilted but still bright green.
8. To taste, add salt and pepper.
9. Serve right away.

60. KETO TORTILLA CHIPS (VEGAN, GLUTEN-FREE)

Prep Time: 10 Minutes | Cook Time: 8 Minutes

Total Time: 18 Minutes | Serving: 30

Ingredients

- 1 tbsp Chia Seeds
- ¼ cup of Water
- 1 cup of Almond Flour
- 1 tbsp Extra Virgin Olive Oil

Spices recommended:

- ¼ tsp Ground Cumin
- ¼ tsp Salt
- ¼ tsp Garlic Powder
- 1 tsp Nutritional Yeast – optional, great for a natural cheesy flavor

Instructions

1. Put it in the oven at 400 degrees Fahrenheit for at least 10 minutes, or 200 degrees Celsius, and cook the contents.
2. Combine the chia seeds with the water in a small basin. Use a spoon to combine. Give it 10 minutes to solidify.
3. In a separate big bowl, combine the almond meal, olive oil, spices, and the chia seed gel from before.
4. Form a dough by combining the almond meal and chia gel with your fingertips. In a minute, you should have dough balls.
5. Flatten the ball of dough using a rolling pin between two sheets of parchment paper.
6. Take off the top layer of parchment paper and Cut the tortilla chips into thin pieces while using a sharp knife or pizza cutter. Triangle chips (tortillas) can be made by shaping rolled dough into a circle. You can reuse the dough to make more chips after you cut around the lid! To make a circle, roll out the dough. If you roll three circles, you'll get 10 chips. Use the pizza cutter to make triangles, just like a round cake.
7. Preheat a baking sheet and place the dough on top.
8. If the color hasn't turned golden brown after 6 minutes, bake for another minute. Fry thin chips for about seven or eight minutes. It takes 8 to 9 minutes for thicker chips. For best results, bake for 6 minutes, stirring once halfway through, to prevent chips from burning.
9. Take them out of the oven and let them cool for 5 minutes on a baking sheet once they're golden brown.
10. The tortilla chips can be easily removed by utilizing a small spatula or knife to cut the parchment paper.
11. Pair with my easy avocado dip or any dip of your choice.

61. PALEO PIZZA CRUST

Prep Time: 2 Minutes | Cook Time: 3 Minutes

Total Time: 5 Minutes | Serving: 4

Ingredients

- 8 large egg whites for thicker bases
- 1/2 tsp baking powder
- 1/4 cup of coconut flour sifted

Instructions

1. Mix eggs/egg whites until opaque in a large bowl. Sift in coconut or almond flour and whisk well to remove clumps. Whisk in the baking powder and mixed spices until combined.
2. Lightly grease a small pan on low heat.
3. Put batter in a hot frying pan and coat well. Put the lid on top of the pan and wait 4 to 5 minutes. until bubbles appear. Flip, cook for 2 more minutes, and remove from pan—watch out, it burns quickly.
4. Use all the batter.
5. Let pizza bases cool. Once cool, poke holes roughly over the top with a skewer for even cooking. A light dusting of coconut flour.

62. PRESERVED LEMON OLIVE TAPENADE

Prep Time: 5 Minutes | Cook Time: 5 Minutes

Total Time: 10 Minutes | Serving: 2

Ingredients

- black pepper, freshly ground
- ¼ cup of extra virgin olive oil
- 2 cloves fresh garlic
- 1 preserved lemon
- 1 tsp preserved lemon juice
- ½ cup of roasted red pepper
- 1 tbsp capers, drained
- 2 cups of pitted, chopped olives
- ¼ cup of fresh cilantro

Instructions

1. Mix all ingredients in the bowl of a food processor.
2. Pulse until well combined and serve with crusty or toasted bread. Enjoy!

63. PALEO CHICKEN YAKITORI SKEWERS

Prep Time: 30 Minutes | Cook Time: 12 Minutes

Total Time: 42 Minutes | Serving: 12

Ingredients

- 2 bundles of scallions, use white & pale green parts only
- Avocado oil
- ½ tsp coarse sea salt,
- ⅛ tsp white or black pepper,
- 1.5pound chicken thighs, boneless, skinless

Instructions

1. Water the bamboo skewers for an hour. After making the teriyaki sauce, let it cool. The remaining 1/4 cup of dressing should be set aside for use as a dip. Cut chicken into 1-inch pieces—season with ½ tsp salt and ⅛ tsp pepper in a large bowl.
2. Scallion slices should be 1 inch. Use only white and pale green.
3. Fold the chicken in half and thread one piece on a skewer, then a scallion segment, on a flat surface. Keep alternating and packing tightly. Each skewer holds 4 chicken slices and 3 scallions.
4. Add 1-2 tbsp avocado oil to a large, preheated skillet. Cook the first side of the skewers for 4-5 minutes over medium heat. Sprinkle salt and pepper on each skewer. Flip and cook for 4-5 more minutes. Add a little salt and pepper. Separate batches and add oil if needed.
5. Gas Grill: Apply avocado oil to the grilling gate, set skewers directly on the grill, cover, and cook, tossing often, for approximately 10 minutes or until chicken is nicely browned and scallions are soft.   Sprinkle salt and pepper 2-3 times while grilling.
6. Using teriyaki sauce, cook skewers for 30 seconds. Turn the skewers again, brush with more sauce, and cook 30 seconds longer.
7. Rest the chicken for 1-2 minutes after removing it from heat. Add more sauce and serve now.

64. HEALTHY ZUPPA TOSCANA

Prep Time: 5 Minutes | Cook Time: 45 Minutes

Total Time: 50 Minutes | Serving: 6

Ingredients

- 1 can of coconut milk
- 1 pound Italian sausage made from below recipe or storebought
- 1 medium white or yellow onion diced
- Salt and pepper to taste
- 4 cups of chicken stock
- ☐½ tsp crushed red pepper flakes
- 2 tbsp garlic minced, about 4 cloves
- ½ bunch kale stems removed
- 4 slices Whole30-compliant bacon
- 4 medium yellow potatoes

- 1 pound ground pork
- 1 tsp onion powder
- 1 tbsp red wine vinegar
- 1 tsp black pepper
- 1 tsp dried basil
- 1 tsp paprika
- 1 tbsp fresh chopped parsley
- 1 tsp red pepper flakes
- 1 tsp garlic powder
- 1 tsp salt
- ¼ tsp ground fennel seed, optional
- pinch dried oregano
- pinch dried thyme

Homemade Whole30 Italian Sausage:

Instructions

1. Combine all of the ingredients for the Italian sausage in a bowl and stir them to combine. Another option would be to brown everything at once in a saucepan while sssssss
2. Place the Italian sausage in a Dutch oven or other medium-sized heavy-bottomed pot and cook over medium-low heat. After that, top it up with some crushed red pepper flakes. Using a spoon, destroy them. Cook until done and golden on both sides. Remove from pan and set aside.
3. Fry the bacon in a spacious oven over medium heat for about 10 minutes or until it's crispy. Separate the bacon pieces and set them aside. Save the bacon fat for later! Then, mix in the garlic and onions. The onions should be tender and translucent after around 5 minutes of cooking.
4. Add the chicken stock to the oven along with the garlic and onions. Get them boiling on high heat. After around ten to twenty minutes, the potatoes ought to be fork-tender. Next, combine the cooked sausage with the coconut milk and reduce the heat to medium. Make sure to heat everything. Toss in the bacon and greens with the soup right before serving. The kale should soften and turn a vibrant green color while cooking—season with salt and pepper to taste.

65. FLOURLESS BROWNIES PALEO

Prep Time: 5 Minutes | Cook Time: 25 Minutes

Total Time: 30 Minutes | Serving: 16

Ingredients

- 6 tbsp tapioca starch
- 1/4 tsp acceptable sea salt
- 2/3 cup of granulated sugar
- 2 large eggs lightly beaten
- 6 TBS Salted Butter or coconut oil
- ¼ cup of unsweetened cocoa powder sifted
- ½ cup of chocolate chips
- cup of chocolate chips
- 2 tsp pure vanilla extract

Instructions

1. Preheat the oven to 350 degrees Fahrenheit.
2. Grease a square pan that is 8 inches by 8 inches. Use parchment paper to line the pan so it's easy to remove if desired.
3. In a tiny bowl, combine the cocoa powder, tapioca starch, and salt by sifting them together. Stack up.
4. Melt chocolate chips and butter in a microwave- or stovetop-safe bowl. Then, give the mixture a good stir until it becomes glossy and smooth.
5. Coat the eggs in the wire whip attachment's bowl and place them in the stand mixer. Beat at a medium-high tempo for one minute. The eggs will be a pale golden hue, and foam will be abundant. Another option is to use a handheld mixer and beat for 60 seconds.
6. Place either granulated sugar or coconut sugar in the bowl of your standing mixer. Continue beating for another minute at a medium-high speed. It may seem thick at first. Another option is to use a handheld mixer and beat for 60 seconds.
7. Melt the butter and chocolate and mix in the vanilla. Beat all the ingredients together to combine them.
8. After adding the dry ingredients, mix until well blended and free of lumps. As you add the half cup of chocolate chips, spread them evenly by hand.
9. Pour the batter into the baking dish. When inserted into a preheated oven, bake for 18–25 minutes or until the surface is firm and a toothpick dipped in moist crumbs emerges.
10. Just a bit longer, at least. Stay warm, or enjoy the chill!
11. Store in an airtight jar in the fridge. To restore its baked-good flavor, simply reheat it in the microwave for 10 seconds.

66. APPLE CRISP (PALEO, VEGAN,

Prep Time: 10 Minutes | Cook Time: 40 Minutes | Total Time: 50 Minutes | Serving: 4

Ingredients

Crisp topping:

- ⅓ cup of whole raw pecans
- ⅓ cup of maple sugar or coconut sugar
- ⅓ cup of whole raw almonds
- ½ tsp Diamond Crystal kosher salt
- ½ cup of unsweetened coconut flakes
- 5 tbsp chilled ghee
- ¼ tsp ground cardamom
- ¼ tsp ground cinnamon
- ½ cup of finely ground almond flour

Apple filling:

- 2½ pounds apples peeled
- 2 tbsp maple sugar or coconut sugar
- 2 tsp tapioca starch
- ½ tsp ground cinnamon
- 2 tsp finely grated lemon zest
- 2 tbsp lemon juice
- whipped coconut topping or ice cream

Instructions

Make the crisp topping:

1. Put the cinnamon, cardamom, maple sugar, salt, almond flour, and maple sugar in a food processor work bowl with a steel blade.
2. The ghee or coconut oil should be cold when you add it. Mix it up five to seven times or until it feels like coarse cornmeal.
3. Add the coconut flakes and nuts. Don't pulse it too much because you don't want to make dough. Pulse it until it looks like wet sand with some nuts in it.
4. Move the topping to a bowl and put it in the fridge for at least 15 minutes to cool down.

Make the filling:

1. Set the oven rack in the middle and heat it to 350°F while the topping chills.
2. Put the apples, maple sugar, tapioca, and cinnamon in a large bowl and mix them.
3. Using a silicone spatula, mix the lemon zest and juice in well.
4. Place the apples in a 2-quart baking pan that is 8 inches square or 9 inches round. Spread them out evenly in the pan.
5. Spread the chilled crisp topping out evenly on top of the apples.
6. The topping should be golden brown after 35 to 45 minutes of baking. Apples should be easy to poke with a fork.
7. Let it cool down for a while. If you want, you can serve it warm or at room temperature and top it with whipped coconut cream or ice cream.

67. PALEO CARROT CAKE WITH ALMOND FLOUR

Prep Time: 30 Minutes | Cook Time:1 Hour

Total Time: 1 Hour 40 Minutes | Serving: 8

Ingredients

For The Almond Flour Carrot Cake:

- ½ tsp Ground Ginger
- ¼ cup of (25g) Toasted, Chopped Walnuts
- 6ounce Carrots, about 2 large, scrubbed,
- ¾ tsp (3g) Fine Sea Salt
- ½ tsp Vanilla Extract
- ¼ cup of (40g) Diced Fresh Pineapple, optional
- 1 tsp Orange Juice freshly squeezed
- ¼ cup of (25g) Shredded Unsweetened Coconut, optional
- ¼ tsp (1g) Baking Soda
- 1 ½ cups of (180g) Almond Flour
- 1 tsp (4g) Baking Powder
- tsp of cream of tartar for the paleo version
- ½ cup of + 2 Tbsp (125g) Coconut Sugar
- ½ tsp Ground Cinnamon
- ¼ cup of (56g) Coconut Oil
- 3 large Eggs at room temperature
- ½ tsp Ground Cardamom
- 3 Tbsp (21g) Ground Golden Flaxseed
- ¼ cup of (40g) Golden Raisins

For The Vegan Cream Cheese Frosting::

- Squeeze of Lemon/Orange Juice about ½ tsp
- ½ tsp Vanilla Extract
- 2 Tbsp (20g) Unsalted Vegan Butter
- ½ cup of (113g) Vegan Cream Cheese
- 2 Tbsp (42g) Pure Maple Syrup

Instructions

To Make The Paleo Carrot Cake:

1. Set a rack in the mid position of the oven and heat it to 350 degrees F. Use 1 tsp of coconut oil to grease a 9-inch cake pan and put parchment paper on the bottom. Mix the ground flaxseed, baking powder, baking soda, salt, cinnamon, ginger, and cardamom with a whisk in a large bowl.
2. Mix the eggs, orange juice, vanilla, and the remaining of the coconut oil in a medium bowl. Use a whisk to make the mixture smooth and silky. Mix the dry and wet ingredients until mixed well. Add the golden raisins, walnuts, and coconut (if using) and mix them in. Add the walnuts, pineapple (if using), and carrots and mix them in.

3. Once the pan is ready, pour the batter into it and smooth the top. For 8-inch pans, bake for an hour. For 9-inch pans, bake for 50 to 55 minutes or until the top is lightly browned, a toothpick inserted in the middle position comes out clean, and the midposition springs back when touched.
4. After 10 minutes, carefully take the cake out of the pan, throw away the parchment paper, and keep it on a cooling rack to cool completely. Put the frosting on top.

To Make The Vegan Cream Cheese Frosting:

1. Beat butter and cream cheese on medium with a handheld or electric mixer until very smooth, about two minutes.
2. Add the vanilla extract, maple syrup, and lemon or orange juice after scraping the sides of the bowl.
3. After about 4 minutes of beating on medium-high, scrape down the sides and bottom [art of the bowl to make it fluffy.
4. For easier spreading, put it in the fridge for 10 minutes if you need to.

68. ONE POT THAI COCONUT CHICKEN CURRY WITH VEGGIES

Prep Time: 10 Minutes | Cook Time: 30 Minutes

Total Time: 40 Minutes | Serving: 8

Ingredients

- 1/2 tbsp ground turmeric
- 1 tbsp coconut oil
- 3 cups of broccoli florets (215 grams)
- 1 can full-fat coconut milk
- salt and pepper, to taste
- 1 1/2 tbsp curry powder, divided
- 2 cups of julienned bell peppers
- for serving: white rice, cauliflower rice, cilantro, lime wedge
- 1 tbsp tomato paste
- 1/2 tsp cayenne pepper
- 1 cup of diced onion (120 grams)
- 1 pound chicken breast
- 1 tbsp Thai red curry paste
- 1 tbsp grated ginger
- 2 cups of cubed sweet potato
- 2 cloves garlic, minced

Instructions

1. On medium heat, warm up a big Dutch oven or a nonstick pot or pan. Please put in the oil and wait 30 seconds for it to get hot. Toss in 1 tbsp of curry powder, ground turmeric, garlic, and ginger. For about 30 seconds, stir the spices around until they smell good and are well mixed. Make sure the garlic doesn't get too hot.
2. Make chicken. Add the chicken, salt, and pepper, then mix the spices with the chicken. Cook for 5 to 7 minutes, stirring now and then, until the outside is golden. If the herbs are getting stuck to the bottom, add a little broth or water. Take it out of the pan and set it aside.
3. Prepare vegetables. Put in the sweet potato, onion, salt, and pepper, and mix everything. To cook for 7 minutes, stir it around a few times. To get the brown bits off the bottom of the pan, add a splash of water or broth. After that, add the broccoli and peppers. Put the lid on top and cook for another 3 to 5 minutes, stirring now and then.
4. Warm-up. Add the cooked chicken, cayenne, salt, pepper, and the last 1/2 tbsp of curry powder. Also, add the red curry paste and tomato paste. Use a stir to mix. I also like to add the chicken juices to make it taste better. Depending on how you want your vegetables cooked, let it simmer for 5 to 10 minutes. As you cook, the curry will get thicker.
5. Have fun! Enjoy it with rice, lime wedges, and cilantro

69. COCONUT CRUSTED CHICKEN TENDERS

Prep Time: 20 Minutes | Cook Time: 20 Minutes

Total Time: 40 Minutes | Serving: 4

Ingredients

- 1/3 cup of tapioca or arrowroot flour
- 2 tsp paprika
- 1/4 tsp cayenne
- 1 1/4 cups of desiccated
- 2 tbsp coconut oil
- 1 1/2 pound boneless
- 3/4 tsp salt
- 2 eggs whisked

Instructions

1. Stir the starch, salt, cayenne, and paprika together in a small bowl or plate until everything is well-mixed. It was icing the eggs together in a different small bowl. Put the coconut shreds in a third bowl or container that is just a little deep.
2. To make your covering go more quickly, arrange the bowls so that the starchy spice mix goes in first, then the eggs, and finally the coconut. Take a big piece of aluminum foil or baking paper and set it away so that you can lay out your chicken pieces as you work.
3. When you dip a chicken piece in the starchy spice mix, make sure to cover all sides well. Shake off any extra starch.
4. The next step is to coat the chicken tender entirely with the egg mixture. Shake off any extra egg.
5. Now, dip the chicken tenders into the coconut flakes and press them into the flakes to cover them well. After coating all of the chicken, put it on the foil or baking paper and set it away while you do it again. As you go, make sure to pack only a few coated chicken pieces at a time.
6. In a big nonstick skillet or pan set over medium-low heat, warm up your coconut oil. To cook the chicken tenders all the way through, add them to the hot oil and slowly fry each side for about 5 to 6 minutes. If you flip your chicken too early or too often, it won't get crispy. Also, make sure there is room between each piece. You may need to work in batches to keep the pan from getting too full. Move the chicken parts to a plate or a rack to cool. Make sure you cook all of your chicken at once. Serve right away and enjoy.

70. MAPLE SHORTBREAD (GRAIN FREE, PALEO, VEGAN OPTION)

Prep Time: Minutes | Cook Time: 18 Minutes

Total Time: 18 Minutes | Serving: 12

Ingredients

- 6 tbsp butter or coconut oil, softened
- 2 cups of almond flour
- 3 tbsp maple syrup, dark grade

Instructions

1. Put melted butter that has been at room temperature into a medium-sized mixing bowl to begin.
2. Using a rubber spatula, mix the almond flour into the butter.
3. Add the maple syrup after the almond flour and butter are well mixed. It's going to be very soft.
4. Place a small amount of cookie dough on a piece of wax paper. Then, roll the paper into a tube that is about 2 inches across.
5. After shaping the cookie dough, put it in the fridge for 4 to 6 hours or the freezer for 1 to 2 hours.
6. Cut the dough into rounds with a sharp knife. This will make about 12 cookies.
7. Warm the oven up to 350 degrees and put parchment paper on a baking sheet.
8. It will take about 15 to 18 minutes of baking until the bottom is golden brow

71. GRAIN-FREE BERRY CRISP

Prep Time: 10 Minutes | Cook Time: 45 Minutes

Total Time: 55 Minutes | Serving: 8

Ingredients

Berries:

- 7-8 cups of mixed berries
- 3 Tbsp maple syrup
- 2 Tbsp arrowroot starch
- 1 Tbsp lemon juice

Crisp:

- 1 cup of almond flour (or almond meal)
- 2/3 cup of shredded or desiccated coconut
- 1 cup of roughly chopped pecans
- 1/2 cup of coconut sugar
- 1/2 tsp sea salt
- 4 Tbsp coconut oil or vegan butter
- 2 Tbsp maple syrup (optional)

Instructions

1. Heat the oven to 350 degrees F (176 C) and put the fruit right into a 9x13-inch or similar dish (I like this one from World Market; change the number and size of pans if you want to make a bigger or smaller batch). Add the lemon juice, maple syrup, and arrowroot on top, and toss everything together.
2. Put the coconut, nuts, almond flour, coconut sugar, and salt in a large bowl. Use a stir to mix. So, add the coconut oil (or vegan butter) and mix it in again, this time with your hands or a spoon, until it's smooth. Check to see if it's sweet enough. Either add more maple syrup or more coconut sugar (I added 2 tbsp (30 ml) more maple syrup).
3. Place the crisp topping on top of the fruit in a thin layer. For 40 to 45 minutes, or until the fruit is popping and the top is golden brown, bake with the door open in the middle of the oven.
4. Wait 10 minutes and then serve. You can eat it plain or with Coconut Whipped Cream or Coconut Vanilla Ice Cream! Cover leftovers and put them in the fridge for up to 4 days.

72. PALEO PUMPKIN MUFFINS

Prep Time: 10 Minutes | Cook Time: 50 Minutes

Total Time: 1 Hour | Serving: 12

Ingredients

For the dry ingredients:

- 2 cups of almond flour or almond meal
- 1 tsp baking soda
- 1 tsp pumpkin spice
- 1 tsp cinnamon
- Pinch of salt

For the wet ingredients:

- 3 large eggs at room temperature
- ¾ cup of coconut sugar
- 1 can 15ounce . pumpkin puree *
- 1 tsp vanilla extract

Topping (optional):

- Handful of pumpkin seeds

Instructions

1. Warm the oven up to 350 degrees. Use parchment paper to line a 12-cup of muffin tin. Put away.
2. Combine all of the dry ingredients in a big bowl.
3. In another basin, mix the wet ingredients.
4. Stir everything thoroughly after adding the wet components to the dry ones.
5. Fill the muffin tin with the batter one-third of the way. Add a few pumpkin seeds to the top of each muffin cup.
6. For even cooking, turn the pan over every 15 minutes or so during the 45–50-minute baking time.
7. Please wait until it's room temperature to serve it.

73. COCONUT JELLY (DAIRY FREE MELO MELO COPYCAT)

Prep Time: 5 Minutes | Cook Time: 15 Minutes

Total Time: 20 Minutes | Serving: 6

Ingredients

- 1 cup of coconut water divided
- 2½ tsp unflavored gelatin powder
- 2½ cups of full-fat coconut milk
- ¼ cup of honey light colored
- ½ tsp vanilla extract
- 1½ cups of sliced fresh fruit optional

Instructions

1. Put ¼ cup of the coconut water into a small bowl. When you add the gelatin, whisk it in well. Put it somewhere else to let the gelatin bloom and get more water.
2. Put the rest of the coconut water, coconut milk, and honey in a small saucepan. Stir the coconut mixture around a lot as you heat it over medium-low heat until the love melts and the coconut milk is hot but not boiling.
3. Take the pan off the heat and add the vanilla and extra hydrated gelatin. Make sure there are no lumps by whisking the mixture.
4. Through a fine mesh sieve into a liquid measuring cup. This will catch any gelatin or honey chunks that still need to melt. Using a mesh strainer, skim off any bubbles that are on top.
5. Then, put the coconut milk mixture into 6 small glass jars that hold 6 ounces each.
6. Put the jars in the fridge without the lids for one hour. Then, put the covers on and chill for another four hours or until the jam is solid. Add fresh fruit on top when it's time to serve!
7. In sealed jars, put the coconut jelly in the fridge for up to three days.

74. KETO BLUE CHEESE BUFFALO CHICKEN BALLS

Prep Time: 10 Minutes | Cook Time: 18 Minutes

Total Time: 28 Minutes | Serving: 6

Ingredients

- 1/2 cup of crumbled blue cheese
- 1/4 cup of chopped celery
- 1/2 tsp sea salt
- 1 large egg
- 1 tsp onion powder
- 1 lb. ground chicken
- 1/2 tsp cracked black pepper
- 2 tbsp water
- 1 cup of shredded mozzarella cheese
- 1 recipe WickedStuffed Buffalo Sauce

Instructions

1. Warm the oven up to 450 degrees F.
2. Put parchment paper around the edges of a baking pan.
3. Add the celery, water, onion powder, salt, and pepper to a large bowl. Then add the chicken, egg, mozzarella, and blue cheese. Mix the things well with your hands.
4. Make about 20 meatballs out of the mixture and put them on the baking sheet as you go.
5. It will take about 18 minutes to bake until the internal temperature is 165 degrees F.
6. Warm up the buffalo sauce in a medium-sized saucepan over low heat at the same time.
7. Run the meatballs through the warm sauce and serve.

75. COCONUT MILK PEPPERMINT HOT CHOCOLATE

Prep Time: 5 Minutes | Cook Time: Minutes

Total Time: 5 Minutes | Serving: 2

Ingredients

- 2 tbsp maple syrup or to taste
- 1/2 tsp peppermint extract
- 1 can | 13.5ounce coconut milk from a can
- 3 tbsp unprocessed cocoa powder

Instructions

1. Put the cocoa powder, maple syrup, peppermint extract, and coconut milk in a small pot on low heat. Use a whisk to mix the ingredients.
2. If you want, you can add your favorite hot cocoa toppings and coconut whipped cream on top. Serve warm. Have fun!

76. MUCVER - CRISPY ZUCCHINI FRITTERS

Prep Time: 10 Minutes | Cook Time: 20 Minutes

Total Time: 30 Minutes | Serving: 12

Ingredients

For the zucchini fritters:

- 4 medium zucchini coarsely grated
- 1 ½ tsp sea salt
- 2 eggs
- 1 tbsp onion powder
- 2 tsp garlic powder
- ½ tsp oregano
- ½ tsp basil
- ¼ tsp pepper
- ½ cup of cassava flour
- avocado oil spray melted coconut oil, butter, or olive oil for the tray

For the sauce:

-
- ½ cup of plain full-fat coconut yogur
- ¼ cup of avocado oil or olive oil
- Juice of ½ lemon
- 1 small avocado pitted
- 2 garlic cloves peeled
- 2 tsp raw honey
- ½ tsp sea salt

Instructions

1. Peel and grate the courgettes. Please put them in a colander and sprinkle some salt on top. Let them drain for 30 minutes.
2. Put the grated courgettes in a tea towel or paper towel that can soak up water. Squeeze out as much water as you can, then move the vegetables to a large bowl.
3. Mix the courgettes with the fresh and dried mint, parsley, dill, egg(s), flour, salt, freshly ground black pepper, and baking powder. Make sure the batter is thick.
4. Put the vegetable oil in a spacious frying pan and heat it over medium heat.
5. When the oil is hot, add a heaping spoonful of the mixture and gently press it down to make it a little flatter. If your pan is big enough, fry four or five cakes at a time.
6. Fry them for a few minutes until they turn golden brown, then use a spatula to flip them over. Fry the other side for a few minutes longer, then put them on a plate with paper towels on top to soak up the extra oil.

77. SATAY BEEF NOODLE SOUP (HỦ TIẾU SA TẾ BÒ)

Prep Time: 3 Hours 15 Minutes | Cook Time: 25 Minutes

Total Time: 3 Hours 40 Minutes | Serving: 6

Ingredients

For The Soup:

- 1 jar Jimmy's sate sauce (360g/0.8lb per jar)
- 20 g / 0.04pound rock sugar (or to taste)
- 1 jar BBQ satay sauce (340g/0.7lb per jar)
- 5 L / 20 US cup of chicken and pork stock
- 1 tbsp chicken bouillon powder
- 1 1/2 tbsp salt (or to taste)
- L / 4.22 US cup of coconut cream
- 1/2 US cup of sesame oil

For The Noodles And Toppings:

- 2 bags of rice noodles
- 1 kg beef (sliced thinly)

Instructions

1. Make stock from chicken and pork. Put in the satay sauces, salt, chicken bouillon powder, rock sugar, coconut cream, and sesame oil. Boil the stock when it's ready.
2. For twenty minutes, let it cook.
3. Important: If you'd like it thicker, let it simmer for longer until it's the consistency you want. Just remember to taste it first and change the flavor to your liking because cooking it longer will change the taste.
4. If you have already cooked the rice noodles, heat a small pot of water and quickly blanch the strands to warm them up.
5. Put the cooked noodles in a bowl to serve. We only serve this one at a time.
6. You can cook some raw beef in the satay soup and then put it on top of the noodles.
7. Add as much soup as you like, and then top with Thai basil, bean sprouts, tomato, cucumber, and a squeeze of lime juice.
8. Enjoy right away as is!

78. PALEO FISH TACOS

Prep Time: 20 Minutes | Cook Time: 6 Minutes | Total Time: 26 Minutes | Serving: 10

Ingredients

Simple salsa (makes 1 ¼ cups):

- 1 whole lime juice or to taste
- ½ tsp coarse salt or to taste
- ½ cup of flat parsley or cilantro, finely chopped
- 2 medium Roma tomatoes, finely chopped
- 3ounce . shallots, , finely chopped

Gluten-free fish taco batter:

- 4 tbsp cassava flour
- 1.5pound firm white-fleshed fish fillets
- 2 tbsp arrowroot or tapioca starch
- 2 large eggs, whisk well
- 1 tsp baking soda
- ¼ tsp ground black pepper
- 1 tsp coarse salt
- ½ tsp smoked or sweet paprika
- 1/2 cup of + 4 tbsp ice-cold sparkling water

Other:

- Shredded cabbage (optional)
- Avocado slices
- 10 pieces 6-inch grain-free Paleo tortilla
- Pineapple cubes (optional)
- 2 tbsp avocado oil

Instructions

1. Salt and tomatoes are all you need to make simple salsa in a bowl. Mix it slowly, cover it, and put it in the fridge until you're ready to use it.
2. Dry ingredients: Put the cassava flour, coarse salt, and other dry ingredients in a large bowl and mix them.
3. Fish: Pat the fish dry gently and cut them into strips that are about 1 inch wide and 3 inches long.
4. Warm up the skillet: Put a big nonstick frying pan over medium-high heat and heat it until it's nice and hot. Put in 2 tbsp of avocado oil.
5. In a separate bowl, whisk the eggs. Then, put them in the bowl with the dry ingredients and mix them. Include fizzy water. Please make sure there are no lumps in the batter by combining it well. It should be like ice cream that has melted.
6. Fry the fish in a pan. Dip it in the batter. Cover it well, shake it off, and then put it in the oil. Depending on how thick the fish is, cook the first side in the pan for about three minutes or until you see a light, thin, golden crust. Do not rush the flip; cook the other side for another

two to three minutes. Please put it on a plate and put it in the oven to stay warm. Separately do this so the pan is manageable.

7. Put the fish fillets on top of the tortillas and decorate them with simple salsa, avocado, pineapple, and shredded cabbage, if you want. It comes with a lime wedge to squeeze.

79. WHOLE30 TUNA SALAD (NO MAYO)

Prep Time: 5 Minutes | Cook Time: 5 Minutes

Total Time: 10 Minutes | Serving: 3

Ingredients

- 2 tbsp tahini
- 2 5-oz cans of wild-caught tuna, drained
- salt and pepper, to taste
- 1/3 cup of diced red onion
- 1 cup of diced red bell pepper
- 1/4 cup of parsley, roughly chopped
- pinch of red pepper flakes
- 1 cup of diced green apple
- 2 tbsp lemon juice

Instructions

1. Put everything in a medium-sized mixing bowl and mix it all. Eat it by itself, in a salad, on a lettuce wrap, or any other way you like! For up to 5 days, keep in the refrigerator in a glass jar with a tight lid.

80. BUFFALO CHICKEN DIP {PALEO, WHOLE30}

Prep Time: 5 Minutes | Cook Time: 40 Minutes

Total Time: 45 Minutes | Serving: 8

Ingredients

- 1 1/4pound chicken tenders
- 1/2 tsp smoked paprika
- 1 tbsp olive oil Plus sea salt and pepper
- 2/3 cup of coconut cream t
- 2 cloves garlic minced
- 1 tsp dried dill
- 1/2 medium onion chopped
- 1 tbsp brown mustard Whole30 compliant
- 1 1/2 Tbsp fresh lemon juice
- 1/3 cup of hot sauce Whole30 compliant - I used Franks Red Hot Original
- 1 tsp onion powder
- 1 tsp garlic powder
- 1 Tbsp ghee or other cooking fat
- 2/3 cup of homemade mayo or purchased paleo mayo

Instructions

1. Warm the oven up to 400 degrees and put aluminum foil on a baking sheet. Spray some olive oil on a baking sheet and season the chicken with salt and pepper. Take it out of the oven and let it cool for 15 to 20 minutes. Turn down the oven to 350 F.
2. In the meantime, put the ghee in a small skillet and heat it to medium heat. Once the onions are soft, put the garlic and stir-fry it for another minute or two. Take it off the heat and set it aside.
3. To make the sauce smooth, mix the mayo, coconut cream, mustard, garlic powder, onion powder, dill, paprika, hot sauce, and lemon juice in a large bowl with a whisk. Get your chicken breasts and shred them. Then, add them to the mix with the cooked onions and garlic.
4. Mix everything, then put it in a small casserole dish. Bake in a 350° oven for 15 to 20 minutes, until the edges bubble and the dip is hot all the way through. Serve hot with vegetables, tostones, or plantain chips you make yourself or as a main dish on top of a baked potato. Have fun!

81. PAN SEARED COD WITH GINGER SAUCE

Prep Time: 10 Minutes | Cook Time: 5 Minutes

Total Time: 15 Minutes | Serving:6

Ingredients

- 1pound Cod Fillet or any white meat fish you prefer
- 1/8 tsp Salt

- 1/8 tsp Black Pepper
- 1 tbsp Cooking Oil neutral, no flavor or taste

Sauce:

- 1 tbsp chopped onion
- 1/2 Inch Ginger
- 3 1/2 tbsp Rice Vinegar, no sugar added version
- 2 tbsp Soy Sauce

- 1/2 tbsp Sweetener, your preferred sweetener
- 1/4 tsp Lemon Zest
- 1/4 tsp Lemon Juice

Instructions

1. Collect all of the materials.
2. To remove any surplus liquid from the fish, dab it with a paper towel., and then season both sides with salt and pepper. Put aside.
3. The onion should be roughly chopped before being tossed into the food processor.
4. Peel the ginger with a peeler. Add the chopped blocks to the food processor after you trim them.
5. Toss the lemon zest into the food processor after using a zester. Toss 1/4 tsp of lemon juice into the food processor using the same lemon.
6. Blend the sweetener, soy sauce, and rice vinegar for 20–30 seconds in a food processor or until the consistency you desire is achieved. When ready, move to a bowl that can be used as a dip.
7. In a cast-iron skillet, heat some neutral cooking oil over high heat until it reaches the desired temperature.
8. Carefully add the cod to the cast-iron pan when the oil is hot; be careful, as the fat will splatter. Reduce heat to medium-high. Depending on the thickness, cook covered for one to three minutes. Hold the meat still while it sears.
9. After 1–3 minutes, carefully turn the fish over, put the lid back on, and cook for another 1–3 minutes.
10. Serve the cod with ginger sauce after carefully transferring it to a serving plate.

82. CAJUN BLACKENED COD

Prep Time: 10 Minutes | Cook Time: 5 Minutes

Total Time: 15 Minutes | Serving: 4

Ingredients

- 2 pounds cod fillets 4 with bones
- 2 tsp chili powder
- 2 tsp cumin powder
- 1 tsp garlic powder
- 1 tsp pepper
- 2 tsp taco seasoning
- 2 tbsp canola oil
- 2 tbsp lemon juice drizzle of lemon juice - optional

Instructions

1. After rinsing, pat dry the fish. I was using paper towels.
2. Mix the chili powder, cumin powder, garlic powder, pepper, and taco seasoning; coat both the top and bottom of the fish.
3. Heat the canola oil in an iron skillet over medium-high heat.
4. Flake the fish quickly with a fork after sautéing it for two to three minutes per size, depending on the fish.
5. Finish off the dish with a garnish and a squeeze of lemon juice. Pair it with a colorful vegetable platter, or stuff it into your go-to fish tacos.

83. PALEO BATTERED FISH

Prep Time: 10 Minutes | Cook Time: 10 Minutes | Total Time: 20 Minutes | Serving: 5

Ingredients

- 2 large eggs
- 1/2 cup of olive oil
- 3/4 cup of tapioca starch
- 1/4 tsp black pepper
- 24 ounces Alaskan cod fillets
- 1/4 cup of sparkling water
- 1/4 cup of coconut flour
- 1 tsp garlic salt
- 1 tsp salt

Instructions

1. A small bowl should be used to mix the tapioca starch, coconut flour, seasonings, eggs, etc.
2. Warm up the pan over medium heat, and then add the, warm up half a cup of olive oil.
3. If the cod fillets are on the large side and you prefer smaller pieces, cut them in half diagonally. To dry the cod fillets gently, use a paper towel.
4. Coat the cod fillets with batter and drop them into hot oil once the oil is hot.
5. Once the fillets have cooked for 4 minutes, carefully turn them over and continue cooking for another 3 to 5 minutes or until the inside is white and flaky. Take care not to cook it for too long.
6. If you want your fillets to retain their crunchiness, use a spatula to lift them out of the oil and set them on a wire rack. Serve right away.

84. SMOKED SALMON, AVOCADO, AND ARUGULA SALAD

Prep Time: 5 Minutes | Cook Time: Minutes

Total Time: Minutes | Serving: 4

Ingredients

- 1 cup of microgreens
- 6 ounces smoked salmon, torn into pieces
- 1 1/2 avocado, sliced
- salt and pepper
- Champagne Vinaigrette
- 1/2 red onion, thinly sliced
- 1 pear, sliced
- 4 cups of arugula

Instructions

1. Pour the Champagne Vinaigrette over the salad after putting all of the ingredients in a bowl. Gently mix everything in order and serve right away.

85. BRAZILIAN FISH STEW (MOQUECA!)

Prep Time: 20 Minutes | Cook Time: 30 Minutes

Total Time:40 Minutes | Serving: 4

Ingredients
Fish:

- 1 – 1 1/2 pounds firm white fish- Halibut
- 1/2 tsp salt
- one lime- zest and juice

Stew/ Sauce:

- 2–3 tbsp coconut or olive oil
- 1 onion- finely diced
- 1/2 tsp salt
- 1 cup of carrot, diced
- 1 red bell pepper, diced
- 4 garlic cloves- roughly chopped
- 1/2 jalapeno, finely diced
- 1 tbsp tomato paste
- 2 tsp paprika
- 1 tsp ground cumin (or whole seed)
- 1 cup of fish or chicken stock
- 1 1/2 cups of tomatoes, diced
- 1 14-ounce can of coconut milk
- more salt to taste
- 1/2 cup of chopped cilantro
- squeeze of lime

Instructions

1. Clean the fish, pat it dry, and then cut it into 2-inch pieces. Could you put it in a bowl? Put in salt, lime zest from half of the lime, and lime juice. Just a little massage will cover everything well. Put away.
2. Put the olive oil in a large sauté pan and heat it over medium-high heat. Salt and add the onion. Cook for two to three minutes. Slow down the heat, then add the jalapeño, bell pepper, carrot, and garlic. Cook for another 4 to 5 minutes. Put in the stock, spices, and tomato paste. Mix, then bring to a low boil and add the tomatoes. Transfer to a medium-low oven and cook, covered, for 5 minutes or until the carrots are soft.
3. Feel free to add more salt if you think it needs it after you add the coconut milk.
4. Place the fish in the stew and simmer it for 4 to 6 minutes or until it's fully cooked. Pour the tasty coconut broth over the fish and cook until it's done the way you like it, or for longer if you want thicker pieces. This can also be finished in an oven set to 350F.
5. Taste, change the amount of salt, and squeeze in some lime.
6. Place the dish on top of rice and top with scallions or cilantro. Squeeze some lime juice over the top.You can put some olive oil if you want.

86. HEALTHY GLUTEN-FREE SALMON PATTIES WITH CHIPOTLE LIME SAUCE

Prep Time: 15 Minutes | Cook Time: 16 Minutes| Total Time: 31 Minutes | Serving: 4

Ingredients

For the Chipotle Mayo:

- ⅔ cup of mayonnaise
- 2 tbsp chipotle pepper salsa
- 2 tsp lime juice
- ¼ tsp garlic powder
- ¼ tsp salt

For the Salmon Cakes:

- 14-ounce can salmon, drained, or 3 5-6 ounce cans
- ½ small onion, finely chopped
- 2 tbsp fresh cilantro, chopped
- 1 large sweet potato, cooked, peeled, and mashed
- 2 large eggs
- ⅓ cup of mayonnaise
- 1 tbsp Creole seasoning or your favorite

Instructions

To make the Chipotle Mayo:

1. In a bowl, whisk together all of the ingredients until the mixture is smooth. Put leftovers in the fridge to cool them down, and then store them in an airtight container for up to a week.

Cakes made with salmon:

1. Warm the oven up to 350F and use cooking spray or oil to grease a 12-muffin pan.
2. Put the salmon, onions, and cilantro in a large bowl and mix them. Add the sweet potato mashed and mix it in.
3. Put the eggs, chipotle mayo, and creole seasoning on top. Mix the ingredients with a large fork or your hands until the salmon and sweet potato are well mixed.
4. Spoon two tbsp of the salmon and sweet potato mix into each muffin cup of that has been greased. Use the back of a spoon to press down.
5. For sixteen minutes, or until a toothpick comes out clean, bake the salmon cakes.
6. Take the pan out of the oven and set it on a wire rack. Take the cakes out of the muffin pan and let them cool for 5 minutes.
7. Put the chipotle mayo on top of the salmon cakes.

87. PALEO SALMON CHOWDER WITH COCONUT MILK (AIP)

Prep Time: 15 Minutes | Cook Time: 50 Minutes

Total Time: 1 Hour 5 Minutes | Serving: 6

Ingredients

- 2 medium turnips peeled and cubed
- small onion chopped
- 1 tbsp apple cider vinegar
- sprigs fresh thyme chopped
- 1 medium carrots sliced
- ½ tsp sea salt. Add more to taste
- ⅔ cup of canned coconut milk
- 32 ounces chicken bone broth
- 2 green onions sliced (optional)
- 4 cloves garlic minced
- 2 tbsp lard or coconut oil
- 3 stalks of celery chopped
- 2 tbsp lime juice or lemon juice
- 1 pound salmon fillet cut into bite-sized pieces

Instructions

1. Use a Dutch oven or a big pot to melt the fat. Fry the onions in the hot fat for about 5 minutes or until they turn transparent.
2. After you add the garlic, keep cooking until the food smells good. Then add the celery, carrots, and turnips and mix them in. After 5 to 10 minutes, the vegetables should have a light brown color.
3. Add the salt, vinegar, thyme, and broth and mix well. Turn the heat down to low, cover, and cook for 30 minutes. This will soften the vegetables.
4. Take out any carrots before putting 2 cups of the soup into a blender. Puree the soup until it is smooth. Blend the mix and add it to the soup.
5. After you add the salmon and coconut milk, keep the pot on low heat until the fish is done.
6. Put lime or lemon juice to taste, and if you want, green onions can be used as a garnish.

88. GARLIC BUTTER BAKED SALMON IN FOIL

Prep Time: 6 Minutes | Cook Time: 20 Minutes

Total Time: 26 Minutes | Serving: 5

Ingredients

- 2 cloves garlic, minced
- ¼ tsp Italian seasoning, red pepper flakes, and black pepper
- 2 tbsp lemon juice and cold butter
- Prevent screen from sleeping
- 1 tbsp chopped parsley for garnishing (optional)
- Hands Free Mode:
- ½ tsp salt
- OnOff

1 ¼ pound sockeye or coho salmon

Instructions

1. Set up: Put a rack in the middle of the oven and heat it to 375oF.
2. Sauce: Put the minced garlic and lemon juice in a saucepan over medium-low heat. Let the lemon juice reduce until it's only 1 tbsp . Take the pan off the heat and swirl it around so the butter starts to melt. After taking it off the heat for a few seconds, put it back on and keep stirring it until the butter melts completely. Please do it again with the second tbsp of butter. Put the Italian seasoning, red pepper flakes, salt, and pepper in the butter once it's all melted. Then, take the sauce off the heat.

3. Bake: Put the salmon filet in a piece of foil that is big enough to fold over and seal. Spread the garlic butter sauce on the salmon with a brush or a spoon. So the sauce doesn't leak, cover it with foil, making sure all the sides are closed. Put the salmon in the oven for 12 to 14 minutes or until it feels firm primarily. Oversee the fish so it doesn't burn while you broil it for two to three minutes with the foil open. Take it out of the oven and sprinkle parsley on top. Serve right away.

89. EASY HOT CRAB DIP WITH CREAM CHEESE

Prep Time: 5 Minutes | Cook Time: 45 Minutes

Total Time: 50 Minutes | Serving: 6

Ingredients

- 6 ounces cream cheese
- 1/2 tsp smoked paprika
- 1/2 cup of slivered almonds
- 1/2 tsp horseradish
- 8 ounces jumbo lump crab
- 1/4 cup of minced scallions
- salt and pepper, to taste
- 6 ounces of full-fat Greek yogurt
- 1/2 tsp garlic powder

Instructions

1. Warm up the oven up to 350 degrees Fahrenheit and put butter in a small baking dish.
2. Mix the ingredients. Put cream cheese, yogurt, scallions, horseradish, garlic powder, smoked paprika, salt, and pepper in a medium-sized bowl. Mix the ingredients well, making sure there are no lumps of cream cheese. To get more pieces from jumbo lump crab meat, break it up a bit. Crab and slivered almonds should be mixed in, but some should be saved to sprinkle on top. Be sure to cover the baking dish with the mix. The word that has been greased. Add the rest of the slivered almonds on top.
3. Bake. Please put it in the oven and bake for 40 to 45 minutes or until it puffs up and turns golden brown.
4. Have fun! Put some thinly sliced green onion on top and serve with bread, crackers, or chips. Have fun right away!

90. EASY GROUND BEEF STIR FRY

Prep Time: 15 Minutes | Cook Time: 15 Minutes

Total Time: 30 Minutes | Serving: 4

Ingredients

Stir fry sauce:

- 3 tbsp low-sodium soy sauce
- 2 tbsp oyster sauce
- 1 tbsp dark soy sauce
- 1 tbsp hoisin sauce
- 2 tsp Chinese cooking wine,
- 1 tsp sesame oil
- 1 tsp white granulated sugar (OPTIONAL)

Stir fry:

- 4 cloves garlic, minced
- 1 pound lean ground beef (mince) (500g)
- 1 tbsp oil
- 1 tsp minced ginger
- salt and pepper, to taste
- 1 small onion, sliced
- 1 large carrot, peeled and shredded
- 1 head cabbage, core removed and leaves shredded

Instructions

1. In a bowl, mix the curry ingredients—reserve sauce for later use.
2. With a large skillet set over medium-high heat, heat the cooking oil. Cook the onion for approximately three minutes or until it starts to soften. After 30 seconds of cooking, the ginger and garlic should begin to smell fragrant.
3. After approximately 5 minutes of browning, add the beef and break it up with the end of a wooden spoon while cooking.
4. After the meat has browned, add half of the sauce and stir-fry until coated.
5. Cook, stirring occasionally, until the cabbage wilts, then add the carrots and cabbage. Add salt and pepper according to taste. Mix in the rest of the sauce. Warm it up before serving.

91. PALEO CHICKEN AND BROCCOLI

Prep Time: 15 Minutes | Cook Time: 20 Minutes | Total Time: 35 Minutes | Serving:

Ingredients

Chicken:

- Sea salt and black pepper
- 2 Tbsp avocado oil or olive oil
- 1/2 tsp garlic powder
- 1 tbsp coconut aminos
- 1/2 tsp onion powder
- 2 tsp arrowroot or tapioca flour
- 1 1/2 lbs boneless skinless chicken thighs

Sauce:

- 6 Tbsp coconut aminos
- 1 tsp sesame oil
- 2 tsp arrowroot or tapioca flour
- 5 Tbsp chicken bone broth

Remaining ingredients:

- 1 large head of broccoli
- 4 scallions sliced
- 4 cloves garlic minced
- 1 inch fresh ginger peeled and minced

Instructions

1. Since the stir-fry will cook in a flash, make sure all of your ingredients are ready to go before you start.
2. Put the broccoli florets in a big bowl and cook them for 2 minutes on high heat in the microwave to make them blanch. Return to the heat and stir for an additional minute or until they become just slightly soft.
3. Add the sliced chicken, arrowroot or tapioca, salt, pepper, garlic, and onion powder, and 1 tbsp of coconut aminos to a bowl and mix well. To dissolve the sauce ingredients, whisk them together in a separate bowl.
4. Put the avocado or olive oil into a big nonstick skillet or wok set over medium-high heat. Arrange the cooked chicken in a single layer once it's hot. Cook for approximately 2 more minutes, or until done, after searing for about 3 minutes. Transfer to a serving platter and depart.
5. Reduce heat to medium and reserve skillet liquids and oil. When the garlic and ginger begin to smell fragrant, add the white parts of the scallions and continue to sauté. Toss in the chicken and broccoli with the stir-fry sauce and coat everything evenly. Just enough time to heat through and blend flavors; the sauce should thicken immediately afterward.
6. Take it off the heat and garnish it with the green part of the scallions. Serve it hot over cauliflower rice. Savor it!

92. THAI BASIL CHICKEN BOWLS.

Prep Time: 10 Minutes | Cook Time: 20 Minutes

Total Time: 30 Minutes | Serving: 6

Ingredients

For the rest of the bowls:

- 1.5 lbs chicken breast
- 1 tbsp fish sauce
- 1 tsp toasted sesame oil
- 1 tbsp avocado oil
- Sea salt and pepper
- 4 cloves garlic, minced
- 2 cups of cauliflower rice
- 1 tsp ground ginger
- 3 tbsp coconut aminos
- 1 tbsp avocado oil

For the chicken:

- 1 onion, cut into thick wedges
- 1 tsp ground pepper
- 1 jalapeño, thinly sliced into rounds, optional

For the sauce:

- 1 tsp arrowroot powder
- 3 cups of Thai/Asian basil (can sub with Italian basil)
- 3 green onions, chopped, (optional garnish)
- 3 small bell peppers, thinly sliced

Instructions:

1. Roll out the chicken breasts to a consistent thickness by using a meat mallet or a rolling pin. Separate the breasts by wrapping them in plastic wrap or parchment paper. Cut into thin strips after that.
2. Toss the chicken with the avocado oil in a big wok or skillet set over medium heat. Add a good amount of ground pepper and sea salt. Ten to twelve minutes of cooking time, stirring once or twice should be enough to cook the chicken through.
3. As it's cooking, prepare the garlic, onion, bell peppers, green onion, and jalapeño according to the instructions and set them ignoring it.
4. In a tiny bowl or jar, whisk together all of the sauce ingredients. Leave aside.
5. After the chicken is cooked, take it out and place it on a plate.
6. While the onions and peppers soften, which should take about 3 to 4 minutes, sauté the bell peppers and avocado oil with the onion wedges in the same skillet over medium heat, stirring occasionally, which should take about 3 to 4 minutes.
7. Garlic, jalapeño (if desired), and basil should be added. Cook for another 1-2 minutes.
8. Return the chicken and sauce to the pot. Just a few minutes in the pan will reheat the chicken, so stir everything together before serving. Top with green onion and serve over white rice or cauliflower.

93. ASIAN GROUND TURKEY AND GREEN BEAN STIR FRY

Prep Time: 10 Minutes | Cook Time: 15 Minutes

Total Time: 25 Minutes | Serving: 4

Ingredients

- 2 tbsp olive oil, divided
- 1pound green beans, trimmed and chopped
- Salt and pepper, to taste
- 1pound ground turkey
- 1/2 cup of onion, chopped
- 3 cloves garlic, minced

For the sauce:

- 1/4 cup of low-sodium soy sauce
- 2 tbsp honey
- 2 tsp chili garlic sauce
- 1 tsp sesame oil
- 1 tsp fresh ginger, grated
- 1/4 tsp pepper
- 1/4 tsp red pepper flakes

Instructions

1. Warm up one tbsp of olive oil in a big pan over medium-high heat. Toss the green beans into the hot pan and season with salt and pepper.
2. After about 6 minutes of cooking, the green beans should be soft but still crisp. They should start to get a little char. We don't want green beans that fall over! Put the green beans in a bowl and set them aside.
3. Toss the chopped onion into the hot pan along with the last tbsp of olive oil. For about two to three minutes, until the onion smells good and is clear, add the garlic. Be careful not to burn the garlic as you add it to the pan and cook for another 30 seconds.
4. Brown the ground turkey until it is broken up and the turkey is done.
5. Mix the soy sauce with the other ingredients., chili garlic sauce, honey, sesame oil, ginger, and spices while the ground turkey cooks in the pan.
6. Put the cooked green beans back into the pan and add the sauce. Please make sure the ground turkey and green beans are well covered with the dressing by mixing them well. Please keep it on low heat for another two to three minutes until the sauce gets thick. Enjoy it with hot rice

94. PALEO BEEF WITH BROCCOLI

Prep Time: 15 Minutes | Cook Time: 10 Minutes

Total Time: 25 Minutes | Serving: 4

Ingredients

- 2 cloves garlic, minced
- 2 pieces thinly sliced ginger, finely chopped
- 1 to 2 heads of broccoli
- 1pound beef
- Ghee or cooking fat of your choice

Beef marinade:

- 1/4 tsp black pepper
- 1/4 tsp baking soda
- 1 tsp arrowroot/sweet potato powder
- 1/2 tsp coarse sea salt
- 1 tbsp sesame oil
- 2 tbsp coconut aminos

Sauce combo:

- 1 tbsp red boat fish sauce
- 2 tbsp coconut aminos
- 1/4 tsp black pepper
- 2 tsp sesame oil

Instructions

1. Cut the beef into thin slices, about ¼ inch thick. Use the ingredients under "beef marinade" to flavor thin slices of beef. Combine well. Put broccoli florets in a container that can go in the microwave. Add one to two tbsp of water. Cover loosely with a lid or a damp paper towel, and heat for two minutes. Broccoli should be soft but still crunchy. Put away.
2. Put a wok on mid-range heat and add 1 ½ tbsp of ghee. Turn down the heat to medium and add the garlic and ginger once it's hot. Add a pinch of salt and stir-fry for about 10 seconds until the food smells good.
3. It's time to add the beef that has been marinated. Spread the beef out evenly on the bottom of the sauté pan. Cook until the beef's edge gets a little darker and crispy. Do the same thing with the flip slide. It should be about ¾ of the way cooked through and have a crispy, charred top.
4. Put in "Sauce Combo." Stir-fry for one minute. Put broccoli in. Stir-fry for another 30 seconds. Toss everything together.

95. WHOLE30 CHICKEN CURRY (LOW CARB, PALEO)

Prep Time: 10 Minutes | Cook Time: 40 Minutes | Total Time: 50 Minutes | Serving: 4

Ingredients

- 2 ½ Tbsp. + 1 tsp. ghee divided
- 1 large red onion diced
- Tbsp. ginger thinly sliced
- 6 cloves garlic thinly sliced
- 1 Tbsp. chili powder
- 2 Tbsp. curry powder
- ½ tsp. turmeric
- ½ tsp. garam masala
- dash cinnamon

- salt to taste
- water as needed
- 1 cup of Roma Tomatoes diced
- 2 large boneless skinless chicken breasts
- 4 cups of mushrooms quartered (about 8ounce .)
- 1 14-ounce can coconut milk
- cayenne pepper to taste

To Serve:

- cauliflower rice steamed
- 1 tsp. ghee
- 1 tsp. mustard seeds

- 2 serrano chiles split
- fresh cilantro leaves chopped

Instructions

1. A giant skillet over medium heat should be heated with 1 1/2 tbsp of ghee. While the ginger is cooking, soften the onions. When the garlic begins to smell, add it and cook, stirring often, for another minute or two.
2. Garam masala, cinnamon, turmeric, chili powder, curry powder, and a few large pinches of salt should be added. After thorough mixing, sauté over low heat for approximately 20 minutes or until the toffee is brown without being burned. To avoid scorching, add a tbsp or two of water as necessary. The curry aroma will become more noticeable as the cooking progresses.
3. Toss in the tomatoes and simmer until the mixture becomes glossy and more soupy than the spice-onion blend. Once taken from the pan, add to a blender or food processor and process until a paste forms. Put aside.
4. Put 1 tbsp of ghee in the skillet and put it back on the stove. Toss in the chicken and cook, stirring often, until opaque throughout. Brown and soften the mushrooms by sautéing them with the addition of the spice.
5. Mix in the curry paste from the third step. After two or three minutes of sautéing, Put in the coconut milk can and half a cup of water. Be sure to mix thoroughly. After the chicken is cooked through and the sauce has thickened, simmer for 10 minutes. Take off the stove.

6. To make the ghee, heat 1 tsp in a small skillet over medium heat. Toss in some green chiles and mustard seeds. While the green chile softens and the mustard seeds begin to pop, sauté the mixture.
7. Before topping with chicken curry and mustard seed-chile mixture, spoon cauliflower rice into individual bowls. Add some fresh cilantro leaves as a garnish.

96. SLOW COOKER ADOBO CHICKEN WITH BOK CHOY

Prep Time: 10 Minutes | Cook Time: 8 Hours 5 Minutes

Total Time: 8 Hours 15 Minutes | Serving: 4

Ingredients

- 4 cloves garlic, smashed⅔ cup of apple cider vinegar
- 1 tbsp brown sugar
- ground black pepper to taste
- 1 bay leaf
- 8 skinless, bone-in chicken thighs
- 2 onions, sliced
- 2 green onions, sliced thinly
- 2 tsp paprika
- ⅓ cup of soy sauce
- 1 large head bok choy

Instructions

1. In a slow cooker, combine the garlic, onions, soy sauce, brown sugar, and bay leaf with the apple cider vinegar. Use black pepper as a seasoning. Top with the chicken thighs. Add paprika to the chicken thighs.
2. Cook, covered, on low heat for eight hours.
3. Turn the slow cooker on high heat. Five more minutes after adding the chicken mixture, stir in the bok choy. Add some green onion as a garnish.

97. BEEF WITH BITTER MELON

Prep Time: 25 Minutes | Cook Time: 10 Minutes | Total Time: 35 Minutes | Serving: 4

Ingredients

- 1 pound beef
- (450g, sliced against the grain

Salt:

- 1 tbsp baking soda
- 2 tbsp oil (divided)
- 6 cloves garlic (finely chopped)
- 2 tbsp black beans (rinsed and drained)
- 1 1/2 tbsp Shaoxing wine

- 2 medium bitter melons

- ½ tsp sugar
- 1 tsp dark soy sauce
- 1 tbsp light soy sauce
- ½ tsp sesame oil
- 1/8 tsp white pepper
- 2 tbsp water

To marinate the beef:

- 1 1/2 tsp cornstarch
- 1/4 tsp baking soda
- 1 tsp oyster sauce

- 1 tsp Shaoxing wine
- 2 tsp light soy sauce
- 2 tbsp water

Instructions

1. First, mix the beef slices with the marinade ((2 cups of water, oyster sauce, Shaoxing wine, light soy sauce, and baking soda). Let the beef sit for 20 minutes.
2. To make the bitter melon, cut each one in half down the middle and scoop out the seeds with a spoon. Clean off all the white parts, as they are the bitter ones. Then, cut the melon into thin slices at a 45-degree angle.
3. Get an ice bath ready and set it aside. Heat the water and Add two tbsp of salt and baking soda. For one minute, blanch the bitter melon. Then, use a slotted spoon to move it right away to the ice bath. Remove the water and set it aside.
4. Set the wok on high heat to warm it up. Put in one tbsp of oil and sear the beef for 45 seconds. Get it out of the wok and put it somewhere else.
5. Slowly add one more tbsp of oil to the wok while it is still hot. For one minute, cook the garlic and black beans. Increasing the heat to high gives the dish the right wok-hay flavor. Next, add the bitter melon and quickly stir-fry it in. Finally, add the sugar, sesame oil, white pepper, dark soy sauce, and light soy sauce. Mix and stir everything well.
6. If you want more sauce, add the beef and chicken stock now. Stir-fry and salt to taste. After this, I like to put a lid on the wok and let the food cook for one more minute. Even though cooking the bitter melon until it's soft won't make this dish look any better, it will taste better and make the bitter melon less painful!

98. EGG ROLL IN A BOWL

Prep Time: 20 Minutes | Cook Time: 25 Minutes

Total Time: 45 Minutes | Serving: 6

Ingredients

- 2 pounds of ground pork
- 2 tsp toasted sesame oil
- ¼ pound shiitake mushrooms stemmed and thinly sliced
- Diamond Crystal kosher salt
- 4 garlic cloves minced
- 1 tbsp ghee avocado oil
- shallots minced
- 1 small Napa cabbage
- 2 tsp rice vinegar
- 2 tbsp coconut aminos
- 1 tsp Red Boat fish sauce
- 2 medium carrots peeled and finely diced
- 3 scallions thinly sliced
- 1 tbsp finely grated ginger

Instructions

1. Heat the ghee in a 12-inch (or more giant) skillet over medium-low heat. Add the mushrooms, carrots, and shallots once it's hot.
2. Put a little salt on top and cook for three to five minutes, until the shallots are soft and the mushrooms can be bent.
3. Stir the food for 30 seconds or until it smells good after you add the garlic and ginger.
4. Break up the meat with a spatula or a wooden spoon.
5. Turn the heat up to medium-high and cook the pork for five minutes or until it is no longer pink.
6. With a slotted spoon, move the cooked pork to a different platter. Do not drain the cooking liquid.
7. Add the cabbage to the pan with a little more salt. Cook for three to five minutes or until the cabbage is soft.
8. Turn the heat down to medium and put the ground pork back in the pan. Use a stir to mix.
9. Add fish sauce, rice vinegar, and coconut aminos to taste. Add more seasoning if you think it needs it after tasting.
10. The pan should no longer be hot. Put a drizzle of sesame oil and a lot of scallions on top to finish. Take a bite and serve!

99. KOREAN BEEF BULGOGI

Prep Time: 10 Minutes | Cook Time: 20 Minutes

Total Time: 30 Minutes | Serving: 4

Ingredients

For the marinade:

:

- 1/4 cup of coconut aminos
- 1.5 tsp coconut sugar
- 1.5 tsp fish sauce
- 1.5 tsp apple cider vinegar
- 1 medium pear, cored and cut into chunks
- 3 cloves garlic, minced
- 1 tsp fresh ginger, peeled

For the rest:

- 1.5 lbs flank steak
- 1 shallot, peeled and diced
- 3 green onions, diced
- 2 tbsp sesame oil
- 2 tbsp sesame seeds

Instructions

1. While you get the other ingredients ready, set the steak aside to marinate. You can also cover the steak and put it in the fridge to marinate for up to 24 hours.
2. Before you cook the steak, do what it says to do with the shallot and green onions.
3. Put the big nonstick skillet on medium heat and add the sesame oil. Add the shallot when the oil is hot. For two to three minutes, stir the food often.
4. Place the beef strips in the pan with the shallot. Pour in any marinade that's still left over. Stir the beef every so often while it's cooking until the marinade juices thicken and start to caramelize. The sauce will cover the beef and make it taste like the sauce overall. After 10 to 15 minutes, when the sauce has reduced enough to coat the meat pieces, take the beef out of the pan. For other cooking instructions,
5. Add sliced green onions and sesame seeds on top and serve right away

100. CHICKEN AND ASPARAGUS LEMON STIR FRY

Prep Time: 5 Minutes | Cook Time: 25 Minutes

Total Time: 30 Minutes | Serving: 4

Ingredients

- 2 tbsp water
- 1 bunch asparagus, ends trimmed
- 1 1/2 pounds skinless chicken breast
- /2 cups of reduced-sodium chicken broth
- 1 tbsp fresh ginger
- tbsp canola or grapeseed oil divided
- 2 tbsp reduced-sodium shoyu
- Kosher salt, to taste
- tbsp fresh lemon juice
- fresh black pepper, to taste
- 6 cloves garlic, chopped

Instructions

1. Sprinkle a little salt on the chicken.
2. Soy sauce and chicken broth should be mixed in a small bowl.
3. Put the cornstarch and water in a second small bowl and mix them well.
4. Set a big nonstick wok over medium-high heat. When it's hot, add 1 tsp of the oil and the asparagus. Cook for about 3 to 4 minutes, until the asparagus is soft but still has some crunch.
5. Place the garlic and ginger in the pan. After one minute, turn the food golden. Put away.
6. Turn the heat up to high and add 1 tsp of oil. Next, add half of the chicken and cook for about 4 minutes on each side until browned and fully cooked.
7. Take it out and set it aside. Please do it again with the rest of the chicken and oil. Put away.
8. Add the soy sauce mix. Cook for about one and a half minutes after it boils.
9. Just before it boils, add the lemon juice. And cornstarch mixture and stir well. Then add the chicken and asparagus back to the wok and mix them well. Take it off the heat and serve.

101. SPICY GROUND TURKEY AND GREEN BEAN STIR-FRY

Prep Time: 5 Minutes | Cook Time: 15 Minutes

Total Time: 20 Minutes | Serving: 4

Ingredients

- 1 lb. green beans
- 4 tsp. coconut oil (or vegetable oil)
- 1 tbsp. sesame oil
- 2garlic cloves, minced
- 2 tbsp. ginger, minced
- 1.33 lbs. 99% lean ground turkey
- 4 tbsp. low sodium soy sauce (GF if needed or coconut aminos for Whole30)
- 2 tbsp. rice vinegar
- 2 tsp. Asian chili garlic paste (like sambal olek)

Instructions

1. Warm the oven up so it can broil. Half of the coconut oil should be added to the green beans. Place on a foil-covered baking sheet. To make it tender and start to char, broil it for 6 to 8 minutes. While it's cooking, shake the pan once.
2. 2At the same time, heat the rest of the sesame oil and coconut oil over medium-high heat. Put the turkey meat, garlic, and ginger in the pan. Brown the turkey until it's done.
3. 3Stir the green beans into the pan after adding them. This is where you add the rice vinegar, soy sauce, and sambal olek. For one minute, cook. If you think it needs more seasoning, add more soy sauce.

103. PALEO CHAR SIU

Prep Time: 10 Minutes | Cook Time: 1 Hour 20 Minutes

Total Time: 1 Hour 30 Minutes | Serving: 8

Ingredients

- 3 tbsp tomato paste
- 1 tsp Red Boat fish sauce
- 2 tsp Diamond Crystal kosher
- 1 tbsp honey, optional
- ½ tsp ground ginger
- tsp Chinese five-spice powder
- ¼ cup of coconut aminos
- 3 pounds boneless pork shoulder roast
- 2 scallions trimmed and sliced thinly (optional garnish)
- ½ cup of plum jam sweetened with fruit juice
- 1 tbsp almond butter creamy

Instructions

1. Fill a small saucepan with water and add the ground ginger, fish sauce, coconut aminos, tomato paste, almond butter, honey (if you're not on a Whole30), and jam. Put in a small saucepan. Let it cool to room temperature. Over medium-low heat, whisk the marinade as it comes to a close.
2. After the sauce is smooth and bubbling, put it in a measuring cup of and let it cool to room temperature. The marinade can be kept in the fridge for up to 4 days and then used when the pork is ready to be roasted.
3. Next, get the pork ready. Make Use of a paper towel to dry the pork. Shoulder dry. Then, cut the meat into 2-inch strips of the same thickness. The pork strips should be about the same size all over. You don't want your char siu to be dry, so it's OK to have fatty pork pieces.
4. Put the kosher salt on all of the pieces of pork. Put the pork in a big bowl or a zippered bag, and pour all but ⅓ cup of the cooled marinade over it. Put the marinade you saved in a container and put it in the fridge.
5. Spread the sauce all over the pork strips with your hands. Put the bowl in the fridge for two to twenty-four hours with a silicone lid or plastic wrap on top.
6. Set the oven rack in the middle and heat it to 350°F. When you're ready to roast the pork, do this. Put the pork on a wire rack that can go on a baking sheet in the oven with a lip around the edge.
7. Put the pork in the oven for 30 minutes and flip the pieces over halfway through (15 minutes).
8. Take the pork out of the oven and raise the temperature to 400°F.

9. Put half of the marinade you saved on top of the pork pieces. Add just enough water to the pan's bottom to make a thin layer and cover it. While the pork cooks, the water will keep the fat from setting on fire.
10. For 25 minutes, roast the pork. After that, flip the pork over and brush it with the rest of the marinade. For another 20 to 30 minutes, or until the pork has a little char on the edges, roast it again.
11. Let the pork rest for 10 minutes, and then cut it into bite-sized pieces against the grain. Put the pork on a serving dish and top it with sliced scallions. Serve! You can freeze food for 4 months or keep it in the fridge for up to 4 days.

104. ASIAN GLAZED DRUMSTICKS

Prep Time: 10 Minutes | Cook Time: 45 Minutes

Total Time: 55 Minutes | Serving: 4

Ingredients

- 8 medium chicken drumsticks, skin removed
- olive oil spray,
- 3/4 cup of water
- 1 tbsp sriracha
- 1/3 cup of balsamic vinegar
- 1/3 cup of low-sodium soy sauce
- 1 tbsp honey, or sugar
- 3 cloves garlic, crushed
- 1 tsp ginger, grated
- 2 tbsp chives or scallions, chopped
- 1 tsp sesame seeds

Instructions

1. Put chicken in a heavy, large saucepan. Spray some oil on it and cook it on high for 3 to 4 minutes.
2. To make the sauce, put in water, balsamic, soy sauce, honey, garlic, ginger, and hot sauce. Cook on high until the sauce simmer.
3. Turn down the heat and let it cook for 20 minutes with the lid on.
4. Take off the lid and raise the heat to high. Let the sauce reduce for 8 to 10 minutes, stirring the chicken now and then until it gets thick. When the glaze starts to get stale, keep an eye on it so it doesn't catch fire.
5. Put the chicken on a plate and cover it with sauce.
6. Put chives and sesame seeds on top and serve.

105.STRAWBERRY POPPY SEED SALAD DRESSING

Prep Time: 5 Minutes | Cook Time: Minutes

Total Time: Minutes | Serving: 6

Ingredients

- salt and pepper to taste
- 1/4 cup of lime juice
- 1/4 cup of olive oil
- 1 Tbsp honey
- 1 tsp poppy seeds
- 1/4 cup of chopped fresh strawberries

Instructions

1. Combined In a blender or small food processor, mix everything but the poppy seeds. Mix it up until it's creamy and smooth.
2. Add the poppy seeds.

106. 5-MINUTE ASIAN SALAD DRESSING

Prep Time: 5 Minutes | Cook Time: Minutes

Total Time: 5 Minutes | Serving: 8

Ingredients

- ¼ cup of extra virgin olive oil
- ¼ cup of seasoned rice vinegar
- 1 ½ tbsp honey (or maple syrup)
- 3 tbsp sesame oil
- 1 ½ tsp soy sauce (I use reduced sodium)
- pinch salt
- 1 -2 cloves garlic minced (optional)

Instructions

1. Mix everything by shaking it.
2. It will last up to two weeks in the fridge.

107. MINT & CILANTRO CHIMICHURR

Prep Time: 5 Minutes | Cook Time: Minutes

Total Time: 5 Minutes | Serving: 8

Ingredients

- ⅓ cup of olive oil
- ½ cup of fresh mint
- salt & pepper to taste
- 3-4 cloves garlic
- ½ cup of fresh parsley
- ¼ cup of white wine vinegar
- ½ cup of cilantro
- pinch of sugar (omit for Whole30/Paleo)

Instructions

1. Put garlic in the food processor bowl and pulse it a few times to make it into small pieces. Pulse the mint, parsley, and cilantro together until they are all chopped up. You might have to stir it a few times to make sure everything is mixed well.
2. Put in the vinegar, red pepper flakes, a pinch of sugar (if you want), olive oil, and salt and pepper. To mix, pulse a few times. Feel free to add more salt and pepper if you like. Please put it in a bowl and serve right away. You can also put it in the fridge in a container that won't let air in for up to two weeks. Have fun!

108. KETO COCONUT FLOUR CHOCOLATE CAKE

Prep Time: 15 Minutes | Cook Time: 50 Minutes

Total Time: 1 Hour 5 Minutes | Serving: 12

Ingredients

- ½ cup of Coconut Flour
- 1 tsp Vanilla Extract
- ½ cup of Erythritol erythritol, Monk fruit, Xylitol
- 2 tsp Baking Powder
- 4 Eggs large
- ½ cup of Unsweetened Cocoa Powder
- 5 oz Coconut Cream

Chocolate ganache.:

- 4ounce Sugar-Free Chocolate Chips
- ½ cup of Coconut Cream or heavy cream

Optional – to decorate:

- 2 tbsp Unsweetened Cocoa Powder

Instructions

1. Warm the oven up to 340°F (170°C). the normal mode
2. Grease a with butter or coconut oil 9-inch round cake pan. Put away.
3. Bring the coconut flour, baking powder, and unsweetened cocoa powder in a medium-sized bowl and mix them with a whisk. Put away
4. You can use any sugar-free crystal sweetener to beat eggs in a different bowl. Using a whisk by hand should take at most 30 seconds. Do it like you're making an omelet?
5. Pour the liquid mix over the mix of cocoa and coconut flour.
6. Add vanilla and full-fat coconut cream (or heavy cream) and mix them well.
7. Mix everything until there are no more lumps, and the batter is shiny.
8. Move the cake batter to the cake pan that has been prepared.
9. Please put it in the middle of the oven and bake for 50 minutes. After 30 minutes, you can put a piece of foil on top of the cake. This keeps the cake's top from getting burned and makes sure the cake cooks evenly inside.

10. Stick a stick into the middle of the cake and remove it clean. This means the cake is done.
11. After 10 minutes of cooling in the cake pan, turn the cake out and let it cool on a rack for at least an hour before adding the chocolate ganache on top.
12. GANACHE CHOCOLATE
13. Get the chocolate ganache ready at the same time.
14. Warm the sugar-free dark chocolate with heavy cream or coconut cream in a medium-sized saucepan over medium-low heat until it starts to bubble up on the side of the saucepan. To keep the chocolate from burning, don't boil the cream and whisk it all the time. After about 3 minutes, it will melt as you work with it, making a smooth, shiny chocolate ganache.
15. Use a piping bag or a squeeze sauce bottle to cover the chocolate cake with the chocolate ganache. If you want, you can decorate with about 2 tbsp of unsweetened desiccated coconut.

109. CHOCOLATE AVOCADO PUDDING (PALEO, KETO)

Prep Time: 5 Minutes | Cook Time: 5 Minutes

Total Time: 10 Minutes | Serving: 4

Ingredients

- 2 medium avocados, soft and very ripe
- ½ cup of unsweetened almond milk
- ½ cup of Hershey's Special Dark Cocoa
- cocoa powder
- 1 tsp SweetLeaf Stevia Drops
- 2 tsp vanilla extract
- ½ tsp instant espresso powder optional

Instructions

1. To make avocados, cut them in half and take out the pit. Then, use a spoon to scrape out the flesh and put it in a food processor. Add the rest of the ingredients.
2. Process everything together until there are no more avocado chunks and the ingredients are well mixed.
3. Spread out in four dessert dishes, cover, and put in the fridge.

110. GLUTEN-FREE VANILLA CAKE RECIPE

Prep Time: 25 Minutes | Cook Time: 35 Minutes | Total Time: 1 Hours| Serving: 12

Ingredients

Dry ingredients:

- 2 1/4 cups of gluten-free
- 3 tsp baking powder
- 1 tsp salt

Other ingredients:

- 1 3/4 cups of sugar 350 grams
- 3 eggs
- 1/2 cup of vegetable oil 100 grams
- 1 tbsp vanilla extract
- 1 tsp lemon juice
- 1/2 cup of sour cream 120 grams
- 1 cup of milk 250 grams

For the vanilla buttercream frosting:

- 1 cup of butter (2 sticks)
- 4-5 cups of powdered sugar
- 1/4 cup of heavy cream or milk
- 2 tsp vanilla extract
- pinch salt

Instructions

1. Warm the oven up to 350F. Prepare two 8-inch round pans or one 9x13 pan with cooking spray. I also like to put a circle of baking paper on the bottom of an 8-inch baker's round pan and grease it again.
2. Mix the salt, baking soda, and gluten-free flour in a medium-sized bowl using a whisk.
3. In the bowl of a stand mixer, put the eggs and sugar. For three minutes, whip on medium-high speed until fluffy and light. Add the oil little by little while the mixer is on a low rate. (Do this slowly so you don't lose the air you've added.) Add the lemon juice and vanilla.
4. Mix on low speed as you add one-third of the dry ingredients. Combine until thoroughly mixed. Please put in the sour cream and mix it in. Mix in another third of the dry ingredients. They are more. After adding half of the milk, add the last third of the dry ingredients. Mix in the rest of the milk. It is complete. (Add the dry ingredients one at a time, followed by the liquid ingredients so that the flour can mix with the batter.)
5. Add the batter to the pans that have been prepared. For 35 to 40 minutes, or until golden and a toothpick stuck in the middle of each cake comes out clean.
6. If you use 8-inch round pans, leave. The cake was to cool for fifteen minutes while still in the pans. Wait 15 minutes for the cakes to cool in the pans. The cakes should then be moved to a wire rack to cool further. Let cool all the way down before frosting.

111. GLUTEN-FREE GULAB JAMUN

Prep Time: 10 Minutes | Cook Time: 15 Minutes

Total Time: 25 Minutes | Serving: 7

Ingredients

For the gulab jamuns:

- 2 ½ cups of white bread crumbs
- ½ cup of cashews
- Vegetable oil for deep frying jamuns
- 2 tbsp chopped nuts

For the syrup:

- 1 ½ cups of water
- 1 ½ cups of sugar
- 8 green cardamom pods
- 1 tbsp lemon juice

Instructions

Make the sugar syrup:

1. In a saucepan, bring the water and sugar to a boil. Set the stove on low, add the cardamom and lemon juice, and cook for five more minutes. Take the heat off.

Make the gulab jamuns:

1. Put the breadcrumbs in a bowl and slowly add the cashew cream while mixing them together. Do this until you have a smooth, soft dough that isn't too dry or stiff.
2. Cut it into 14 pieces of the same size, and roll each one into a ball. You want a ball that is very smooth and doesn't have any cracks that you can see. Grease your hands with oil to make it easier to shape the jamuns.
3. In a fryer, heat the oil. The oil should be around 300 degrees, not too hot. The jamuns won't cook all the way through if the oil is too hot. The outside will brown very quickly.
4. Now, add the jamuns to the fryer or wok a few at a time so they don't get crowded. The oil shouldn't bubble too much. Do not let the jamuns fall to the bottom. Keep moving them around with your spider or a slotted spoon until they turn a deep red color.
5. Place them on a plate that has been lined with paper towels. To make holes all around the jam, use a very thin pin or needle while it is still warm but not hot. This will help the syrup stick to it better.
6. While the syrup is still warm but not very hot, put the jamuns in it. They need to be completely submerged. Let them sit for three hours before you serve them so the syrup has time to soak in.
7. If you want, you can serve jamuns with a drizzle of syrup and a sprinkle of nuts.

112. PALEO CHOCOLATE CAKE WITH PALEO CHOCOLATE FROSTING

Prep Time: 2 Hours| Cook Time: 30 Minutes

Total Time:2 Hours 30 Minutes | Serving: 16

Ingredients

- 1 tbsp pure vanilla extract
- 3 cups of packed blanched fine almond flour
- 1 tbsp apple cider vinegar
- 4 large eggs, at room temperature
- 1/4 cup of coconut flour
- 2 tsp baking soda
- 3/4 cup of virgin coconut oil
- 1 cup of unsweetened almond milk
- 3/4 cup of unsweetened cocoa powder
- 1 batch of Paleo chocolate frosting
- ½ tsp salt
- 1 3/4 cup of coconut sugar

Instructions

1. Heat the oven to 350 degrees F. Put rounds of parchment paper around the bottom of three 8-inch or three 6-inch round cake pans. Spray cooking spray that doesn't stick on the pan and the parchment paper. Paper that isn't made of wood or paper will make the cake stick. Do not forget.
2. To start, use this recipe to make your frosting.
3. Cool the coconut oil and add it to a large bowl. Then, add the eggs, vanilla, apple cider vinegar, and mix the mixture until it is smooth. After adding the almond milk, beat the mixture again until it is well mixed in.
4. Blend the cocoa powder, coconut flour, baking soda, and salt in a different bowl. Incorporate the dry components into the liquid ones. Combine the dry and wet ingredients; stir to combine. Well, after adding them. The mixture will be pretty thick.

5. Split the batter evenly between the pans. Use a spatula to spread it out or in a gentle swaying motion to smooth the top of the batter. For eight-inch pans, bake for twenty to thirty minutes. For six-inch pans, bake for twenty to thirty-five minutes or until a tester comes out clean with only a few crumbs attached. Make sure to turn the pans over every half hour while they're baking.
6. For 15 minutes, let the cake cool in the pan. Then, move it to the fridge to finish cooling. Put the cake in the refrigerator to cool for at least an hour before taking it out of the pan and

frosting it. Before frosting, the cake should be at room temperature. That's very significant. For those who want to, you can make the cake the day before!

7. The frosting is now ready: Take the chocolate coconut cream frosting that has set and put it in a large bowl. For a nice fluffy frosting, use a hand mixer or a KitchenAid mixer to beat it until it forms peaks. Utilize it right away!
8. Place cake layers on top of each other, leaving about 1/3 to ½ cup of frosting between each one. Cover the top and sides with the remaiming of the frosting. Suitable for 12 to 16 people! It's best to put a cake in the fridge after the first day or two of keeping it at room temperature.

113. PALEO PIE CRUST

Prep Time: 15 Minutes | Cook Time: 15 Minutes

Total Time: 30 Minutes | Serving: 1

Ingredients

- 1 ¼ cup of tapioca flour approx. 160 grams
- ¼ cup of coconut flour approx. 24 grams
- ¼ tsp salt
- ½ cup of cold butter 1 stick of cold ghee, cut into pieces
- 1 egg

Instructions

1. Utilize a food processor to mix the flour and salt. Salt together. Once a dough has formed, add the egg and butter and continue to mix. Everything will happen in the food processor.
2. Put the dough in a 9-inch pie dish and press it down.
3. On one hand, bake at 350F for 15 minutes or until golden brown. On the other hand, put a filling inside the pie and bake it according to the recipe (for example, this pecan pie needs 45 minutes)

114. PALEO CHOCOLATE CHIP COOKIES

Prep Time: 10 Minutes | Cook Time: 8 Minutes

Total Time: 18 Minutes | Serving: 19

Ingredients

- ¼ tsp sea salt
- ⅓ cup of dark chocolate chips
- 2 tsp vanilla extract
- ½ tsp baking soda
- ¼ cup of coconut oil, melted
- 2 cups of almond flour
- ¼ cup of pure maple syrup (at room temperature)

Instructions

1. Warm the oven up to 350oF and put parchment paper on a baking sheet, which will help prevent things from sticking.
2. Mix the coconut oil, maple syrup, salt, baking soda, and vanilla extract with the almond flour in a medium-sized bowl. After a good stir, add the chocolate chips and fold them in.
3. To put the batter on the baking sheet that has been prepared, use a 1-ounce cookie scoop or a tbsp . Press the cookies down and shape them however you like with your fingers. They won't spread when they're baked, so make them the shape you want.
4. For 8 to 9 minutes, or until the edges are just beginning to turn golden, bake at 350ºF. There will be more crunch the darker they get.
5. Leave the cookies on the pan to cool for 10 minutes. Then, serve cool or warm. Put these cookies in a container that won't allow air in. Please put it in the fridge for up to two weeks or the freezer for up to three months. If you leave them out at room temperature, they will get soft, so keep them cold for the crispiest results.

115. DOUBLE CHOCOLATE BANANA BREAD

Prep Time: 5 Minutes | Cook Time: 45 Minutes

Total Time: 50 Minutes | Serving: 12

Ingredients

- 2 tsp baking powder
- 1/4 cup of milk of choice
- 1/2 cup of sugar of choice: white, brown, coconut, or sugar-free
- 1 tsp vanilla extract
- 1/4 tsp salt
- 1/4 cup of coconut oil melted
- 2 1/4 cups of gluten-free rolled oats
- 1/2 cup of mashed bananas, approximately 4 medium bananas
- 1/2 cup of cocoa powder

Instructions

1. Warm the oven up to 350F/180C. Put parchment paper around the edges of a loaf pan and set it aside.
2. Put the rolled oats in a high-speed Use a blender or food processor to make them very fine. Very fine.
3. Put your mixed oats, cocoa powder, sugar of your choice, salt, and baking powder in a large bowl. Be sure to mix the ingredients well. Except for the chocolate chips, When you add the last few things, mix them in until everything is smooth. Mix in the chocolate chips.
4. The chocolate banana bread batter should be put into the pan that has been lined. It should be baked for fifty to sixty minutes, or "just" until a skewer stuck in the middle comes out clean.
5. Take it out of the oven and let it cool in the pan for a full hour before cutting it into pieces.
6. HOW TO USE A BLENDER OR FOOD PROCESSOR
7. Warm the oven up to 350F/180C. Put parchment paper around the edges of a loaf pan and set it aside.
8. Everything but the chocolate chips should be put into a blender or food processor. Blend or process until smooth and well-mixed. Mix in the chocolate chips.
9. Put the dish in the baking bake in the oven for half an hour to an hour and a half, or until a skewer inserted in the center emerges almost clean.
10. Take it out of the oven and let it cool in the pan for a full hour before cutting it into pieces.

116. COOKIE DOUGH.

Prep Time: 10 Minutes | Cook Time: 20 Minutes

Total Time: 30 Minutes | Serving: 4

Ingredients

- 1 tbsp pure vanilla extract
- 5 tbsp pure maple syrup ¼ cup of + 1 tbsp
- 1 cup of almond flour
- 2 large pinches sea salt
- ¼ cup of coconut flour
- ¼ cup of dairy-free chocolate chips
- 3 tbsp refined coconut oil melted

Instructions

1. You will not be able to use any other gluten-free (or gluten-containing) flours in place of the flours called for in this recipe.
2. The crust's texture will be affected if you swap out the blanched almond flour for almond meal.
3. Ghee is another suitable alternative to the coconut oil in this recipe.
4. Avoid pumpkin pie filling and go straight for pumpkin puree. Filling, so use canned pumpkin instead.
5. Leave out the extra salt from the pecan pie topping if you're using salted pecans.
6. Storage Reminder: These bars are best enjoyed within three to four days when kept lightly covered for later Use.
7. The bars can be frozen for up to a month after they have cooled entirely. Be careful to keep them in an airtight container, though. Leave to thaw in the fridge for at least one night prior to consumption.
8. Recommendation: Let these bars chill in the fridge for at least four to six hours, or even overnight, for the best flavor. Garnish with a generous dollop of coconut whipped cream and serve chilled.

117. PALEO PUMPKIN PECAN PIE BARS

Prep Time: 20 Minutes | Cook Time: 1 Hour

Total Time:1 Hours 20 Minutes | Serving: 12

Ingredients

Shortbread Crust:

- 1 ¼ cup of Almond Flour
- tsp Baking Soda
- 1 cup of Coconut Flour
- 1 tsp Vanilla
- ½ cup of Coconut Oil melted
- 1 Large Egg
- ½ cup of Pure Maple Syrup

Pumpkin Custard Layer:

- 1 ½ tsp Pumpkin Pie Spice
- ¾ cup of Coconut Sugar
- 2 Eggs
- 1 ½ cup of Canned Coconut Cream
- 15ounce . Can Pumpkin Puree, not pumpkin pie filling

Pecan Pie Topping:

- 1 Tbsp Coconut Oil or Ghee melted
- 1 ½ cup of Pecans finely chopped
- ½ cup of Coconut Sugar
- ⅓ cup of Honey
- ½ tsp Salt

Instructions

1. Flour from almonds, coconut, and baking soda should be mixed in a medium-sized basin. Toss in the coconut oil, egg, syrup, and vanilla, and stir with a spatula or wooden spoon until a thick dough forms.
2. Roll out the crust dough using your hands and press it evenly into a parchment-lined pan. (Hint: moisten your hands to spread the dough if it's too sticky.)Sear in a 350°F oven that has been preheated for fifteen minutes.
3. In a medium-sized bowl, combine all of the custard ingredients and mix with a handheld mixer until smooth. Set aside while the crust bakes.
4. Take the pie crust out of the oven and top it with pumpkin custard.
5. Preheat oven to 350 degrees Fahrenheit or until custard thickens and is jiggly in the middle (a little sticky is OK).
6. In a small bowl, combine all of the topping ingredients and mix thoroughly using a fork to make the pecan pie topping.
7. Carefully remove the pumpkin pie bars from the oven and top the custard layer with the pecan topping. Insert the pecans into the pumpkin mixture very delicately.

8. Place the pan back in the oven and bake at 350F for another 12 minutes.
9. Take it out of the oven and let it cool in the pan for half an hour.
10. After it has cooled completely, please put it in the fridge for at least four to six hours or overnight. Then, cut it into twelve bars and serve them chilled.
11. If preferred, garnish with non-dairy whipped cream. Enjoy

118. NO-BAKE VEGAN CHOCOLATE PEANUT BUTTER CHEESECAKE

Prep Time: 15 Minutes | Cook Time: 2 Hours Minutes

Total Time: 2 Hours 15 Minutes | Serving: 10

Ingredients

Crust::

- ½ cup of raw pecans
- ½ cup of dates pitted (don't forget to remove the pits)!!
- 1 ½ TBS unsweetened cocoa powder
- 2 TBS unsweetened, shredded coconut
- 1 TBS honey or pure maple syrup
- ¼ tsp sea salt

Filling:

- 1 cup of roasted, unsalted cashews soaked for at least 1 hour
- 6 TBS pure maple syrup
- ¼ cup of coconut oil melted
- ¼ cup of unsweetened chocolate or semisweet chocolate chips,

melted:

- ¼ cup of creamy peanut butter
- ½ cup of coconut cream
- 1 tsp pure vanilla extract
- 2 TBS unsweetened cocoa powder
- ¼ tsp sea salt

Chocolate peanut butter topping:

- ¼ cup of semisweet chocolate chips
- 2 TBS creamy peanut butter

Instructions

1. Start by immersing 1 cup of cashews in boiling water until they are entirely covered, which should take at least an hour. Rinse and drain after 1 hour, then continue with the recipe as directed.
2. Roll out the crust by lining a 6-inch deep round cake pan with parchment paper. Put aside.
3. Combine the pecans and dates in the Vitamix blender's container or a food processor using the "S" blade. Blend or process until the mixture is uniform in texture and suggests a coarse meal.
4. Blend or process the remaining ingredients until they begin to form small clumps in the blender or food processor. Be careful not to overprocess the mixture, as it will result in oily bites.
5. After getting the pan ready, pour in the mixture and press it down evenly.
6. Put the crust-lined pan in the fridge while you whip up the filling.
7. Filling: Melt the peanut butter, chocolate, maple coconut oil, syrup, and a small skillet over medium heat medium-low heat or in a microwave-safe dish until smooth. Put aside.
8. In the Vitamix blender's container, combine the cashews that have been soaked, rinsed, and drained with the coconut cream. Mix until combined.
9. Blend or Vitamix the peanut butter and coconut oil mixture with the melted chocolate, vanilla extract, cocoa powder, and salt. Until completely smooth, blend for 30 to 60 seconds. Sometimes, you have to pause, scrape down the sides, and keep going with the blender.
10. After the pan is ready, pour in the filling and spread it out evenly over the crust.
11. After removing the pan from the fridge, return it there for another hour or two to allow it to solidify.
12. For the topping, combine 2 tbsp of peanut butter with 1/4 cup of chopped semisweet chocolate or chocolate chips and mix until thoroughly combined. Distribute evenly over the rigid filling. Let it set in the fridge again.
13. Take it out of the refrigerator and let it rest for twenty minutes before cutting into it. Allowing it to sit at room temperature for a bit improves its flavor compared to eating it straight from the refrigerator.

119. KETO FRUIT DIP WITH ONLY 4 INGREDIENTS

Prep Time: 10 Minutes | Cook Time: 30 Minutes

Total Time: 40 Minutes | Serving: 1

Ingredients

- ⅓ cup of Powdered Erythritol, not crystal
- 1 ¼ cup of Heavy Cream
- 1 tsp Vanilla Extract
- ¼ - ½ tsp Marshmallow Stevia Drops
- 8ounce Cream Cheese softened

Instructions

1. When the cream cheese is soft, add vanilla extract to 1/4 cup of heavy cream, powdered erythritol, and marshmallow stevia drops if you want to. Mix the ingredients well in a large bowl. On medium speed, beat for about one minute or until fluffy and well mixed.
2. Put it aside while you whip the rest of the heavy cream.
3. Put the last cup of heavy cream into a different large mixing bowl. Then, whip the cream with an electric beater until a soft peak forms.
4. Put the whipped cream in the bowl with the cream cheese and mix it in.
5. Gently mix until the mixture is fluffy. Please put it in the fridge for 30 minutes before serving it with your favorite keto fruits.
6. HOW TO STORE
7. Keep in the fridsge for up to 4 days in a container that won't let air in.